Bedside Logic in Diagnostic Gastroenterology

Bedside Logic in Diagnostic Gastroenterology

James Christensen, M.D.

Professor
Division of Gastroenterology-Hepatology
Department of Internal Medicine
University of Iowa College of Medicine
University of Iowa Hospitals and Clinics
Iowa City, Iowa

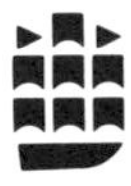

Churchill Livingstone
New York, Edinburgh, London, Melbourne 1987

Library of Congress Cataloging-in-Publication Data

Christensen, James, date —
Bedside logic in diagnostic gastroenterology.

Bibliography: p.
Includes index.
1. Gastrointestinal system—Diseases—Diagnosis—Decision making. 2. Medical logic. 3. Physical diagnosis. I. Title. [DNLM: 1. Gastrointestinal Diseases—diagnosis. 2. Logic. 3. Medical History Taking. WI 100 C554b]
RC803.C475 1987 616.3'075 87-5136
ISBN 0-443-08518-8

Distributed in the United Kingdom by Churchill Livingstone, Robert Stevenson House, 1-3 Baxter's Place, Leith Walk, Edinburgh EH1 3AF, and by associated companies, branches, and representatives throughout the world.

Accurate indications, adverse reactions, and dosage schedules for drugs are provided in this book, but it is possible that they may change. The reader is urged to review the package information data of the manufacturers of the medications mentioned.

Acquisitions Editor: *Toni M. Tracy*
Copy Editor: *Miki Magome*
Production Designer: *Melanie Haber*
Production Supervisor: *Jocelyn Eckstein*

Printed in the United States of America

First published in 1987

To

E. Mott Davis, an archeologist who taught me that details are important,

A. Lawrence Bennett, a physiologist who showed me that the question of function is the focus of all biological inquiries,

James A. Clifton, a gastroenterologist who helped me learn to talk with patients, and

William B. Bean, a medical scholar from whom I learned what scholarship entails.

PREFACE

This book discusses the use of logic in the interpretation of clinical information obtained from interviewing and examining patients for accurate diagnosis in gastroenterology.

Gastroenterology now is much more complex than it used to be. This complexity arose from the explosion in our knowledge of the functions of the gut and its appendages, from our greater understanding of derangements of these functions, and especially from the sophistication and power of contemporary diagnostic techniques. Our predecessors in gastroenterology relied heavily on bedside logic for guidance in diagnosis and on the knife for confirmation. Increasingly diagnostic confirmation relies on laboratory investigation. The directness and accuracy of laboratory investigation make "tests" seductive to the point that they often seem to be applied without the guiding force of bedside logic.

The use of bedside logic to suggest possible diagnoses is both the beginning and the end of the diagnostic process. It is the beginning because it guides subsequent steps to diagnosis; it is the end because the ultimate diagnosis should account fully for the clinical presentation.

Bedside logic is difficult and laboratory investigation is easy. Bedside logic is cheap and laboratory investigation is expensive. The full application of bedside logic can go far to increase the accuracy and reduce the cost of diagnosis in gastroenterology.

Gastroenterology carries a very large body of information in the form of bedside logic. This information continues to be taught (though less than formerly, I think), but almost entirely at the bedside. Skill in bedside logic is assumed to develop mainly with bedside experience but few physicians may soon get the necessary breadth of experience—it takes time and patience to learn by experience alone. Since skills in bedside logic exist, they can be codified to be learned systematically. That is the idea behind this book.

Bedside logic has not been entirely neglected in textbooks of medicine and gastroenterology. In most cases, however, the information is disseminated as elements of what are really encyclopedias, expository accounts organized in terms of nosologic entities. The practical importance of bedside logic, and its strength, tend to be eclipsed in standard textbooks.

I have tried to organize the logic of the diagnostic process in gastroenterology, interpreting symptoms and signs in terms of structure and function rather than defined diseases. Defined diseases, clinical or nosologic entities, are relegated to a minor place—they are really only convenient terms used to define functional derangements that commonly occur together. Such encapsulation is useful as a clinical shorthand but it stereotypes diseases and keeps us from thinking about diseases as processes.

Readers of this book should not expect to find discussions or even definitions of defined clinical entities. I refer to many, assuming that readers will know them. Likewise this book is not a textbook of gastrointestinal physiology. There are many such texts and I assume that the readers have a grounding in that subject. Also, this book is not intended to be a guide to the use and interpretation of laboratory and radiographic observations similar to many conventional textbooks.

I have instead tried to organize information that a gastroenterologist obtains from talking with patients about their symptoms and examining them and to show how this information can point to the organs or the physiologic functions that need to be investigated.

Experienced clinicians know a great many details about the interpretation of symptoms in physiologic terms but they give certain features of a symptom far more weight than they do others. That is, some features are far more important than others. The major features provide major signposts on the road to diagnosis; the others are supportive. Such major features of a symptom can be used to construct algorithms. I have made such algorithms for each symptom except abdominal pain. Pain is far too complex for such treatment. These algorithms appear at the end of each chapter in the form of *decision wheels.*

There are few absolutes in bedside logic. Symptoms vary because of the many variables in how people perceive themselves and their sensations, in what they know as normal, in what expectations they have, and in how they are put together. I constructed the algorithms with much hesitation for such diagrams imply a rigid and simple structure. Still, symptoms fall into patterns that can quickly lead to the right diagnostic path. But remember that these patterns are only averages susceptible to all kinds of exceptions.

You will find a good deal of repetition in this book. This is unavoidable because each chapter is written to stand by itself as a discussion of each symptom when it is the principal symptom. Because all of these symptoms may also appear as secondary or associated symptoms, I found it necessary to discuss them in that light in other chapters. Such repetition, of course, serves to reinforce certain important concepts.

The information contained in this book is compiled from my personal experience and that of many colleagues with whom I have long collaborated or who have written before me. Some previous texts that deal with the general subject are listed at the end of the book.

Some readers may not fully agree with all that is said here and some may be surprised or disappointed that some points have been left out. I have tried to set down systematically a complete and accurate presentation of bedside logic in gastroenterology as I and my associates apply it. I do not pretend to know it all or to have experienced everything.

I offer this text in the hope that it will instruct the novice and inspire the practitioner of gastroenterology to use and develop skill in what is sometimes thought of as part of the art of medicine. I hope that readers will come to regard bedside logic not as an art but as an integral part of the scientific practice of gastroenterology.

James Christensen, M.D.

CONTENTS

Bedside Logic in Diagnostic Gastroenterology

1

TALKING WITH PATIENTS

INTRODUCTION

Diagnosis in gastroenterology rests mainly on what you learn from listening to and talking with a patient about his illness. The process of obtaining an account of that illness—commonly called "taking the history"—is most productive if you treat it as a conversation. As in most conversations, the process works best if discourse is friendly, takes place between people who respect each other, is unhurried, and has a focus or direction.

SOME TACTICS IN PREPARING FOR THE CONVERSATION

A clinical conversation rarely starts out easily. The patient wants help and understanding but he may be impeded by unexpressed fears or guilts. The physician wants information but he may be impeded by haste or distractions. You, the physician, normally control the conversation and it is your responsibility to minimize such impediments.

You can achieve this by several simple maneuvers. These may seem to be no more than common sense and courtesy (as indeed they are) but it is surprising how often they are neglected.

Arrangement of the Conversants

You should see to it that you and the patient are situated in the position that is normal in people who are talking seriously with each other. This means that you must both be seated comfortably with your heads at the same level. When one conversant's head is far above the other's it implies a dominance that can inhibit easy talking. People who are conversing as equals rarely talk face-to-face, with their faces parallel. Such a position is associated with confrontation, interrogation, interview, and intimate conversation but not with formal conversation. A slight obliquity in the faces of the participants is natural and important. Conversations are rarely easy over barriers like desks and tables. The participants should be separated only by empty space. The amount of space is important—

about 3 to 6 feet seems right. More or less separation of the participants impedes good conversation.

These important arrangements can be established by the positions of tables and chairs in the examining room. At the bedside they must be improvised. When the patient is recumbent you should raise his head to about 45 degrees, if that is possible. You should sit down to put your head close to the level of that of the patient. Do not recline in the reclining chair that is often found in hospital rooms. It is better to sit on a low stool. It is not at all bad manners for you to sit on the edge of a bed: It imparts a familiarity and informality that can facilitate conversation.

The Presence of Other People

The clinical conversation is essentially one-on-one, and it normally involves matters that the patient may consider private, so other people should usually be excluded from the room. When patients request that another person be present you should honor the request; relatives can be helpful in adding or confirming elements of the history. In such a case you should not hesitate to arrange for a later interview with the patient alone to clear up specific points if you think that is necessary.

In teaching hospitals, the presence of students, who are strangers to the patient, may impede communication. This problem can be reduced if you introduce these people and explain the reason for their presence. You must always ask permission for the presence of such neutral observers (it is rarely denied). If you sense that observers are significantly interfering with the conversation you should ask them to leave. As in the case when relatives are present you may want to arrange for a subsequent interview alone.

Who is in Charge?

Conversations usually involve peers but only rarely is a conversation fully equally shared. In most conversations one of the participants leads the conversation. Leadership normally falls to the participant who initiated the conversation or to the one who is acting as host. In "taking a history" you are the host and the leader of the conversation and you should carefully maintain that position.

Several simple maneuvers can establish the guest–host relationship at the outset of the interview. It works well to have the patient brought to the examining room by a neutral person, one who is not involved in the interview, so that you enter the room after the patient has. You introduce yourself and shake hands. If other people that you don't know are present, shake hands with them too. These formalities are not trivial, for they signify that you take the process seriously. The question of the presence of observers should be settled at once—it may not need to be asked about, for the wishes of the patient or the other people present may become immediately evident.

THE ELEMENTS OF THE CONVERSATION

The Opening Conversation

After you are seated you should begin the conversation in such a way as to indicate that you are not in a hurry. To do this it is useful for you to make some trivial observation about the weather or anything else that seems appropriate, but a single exchange of trivial remarks is enough. You should then lead to the matter of concern by asking the patient an open-ended question indicating that you want to know why he has come.

The phrasing of this opening question is important, for it may shape the whole subsequent conversation. If you don't know why the patient has come, ask "What can I do for you?" If you already have an idea of the nature of the complaint bring that up at once by forming your question appropriately. If you ask the usual neutral question when you already know the general complaint, you risk making the patient, who usually knows if you already have some preliminary information, think that you are forgetful or distracted. If you know anything at all of the reason for the visit, make it clear at the beginning that you know or remember at least a little.

Once you have indicated that you expect the patient to tell his story most patients will launch some kind of an account of the illness. This is occasionally quite long and detailed, but it is usually brief or incomplete. Some people will ramble off course. If this happens you should interrupt, picking up the thread of the story and getting the patient back on course.

My teachers used to tell me to "let the patient tell his story—that is the present illness." In gastroenterology, at least, this is almost never true. Patients will rarely volunteer to you all you need or want to know. Usually this opening account will give only a general idea of the major complaint with an incomplete chronology. Bedside logic requires far more information than most patients volunteer. They cannot be expected to know what may be important to you. You should allow the patient to complete the opening statement as far as he seems to want to go, for it will contain at least the skeleton of the present illness. Let him finish what he has to say. The flesh of the present illness must be obtained in a subsequent part of the conversation, the Middle Conversation.

The Middle Conversation

The Middle Conversation is impossible to describe or to dictate, since it must be shaped to fit each case, but three general principles are often neglected.

First, you must maintain a normal degree of eye contact with the patient as you would do in any other focused and personal conversation. Second, you must never take notes in the Opening and the Middle Conversations. Note-taking converts a conversation into an interrogation and it makes the patient think that you aren't interested enough to try to remember his story, even for a brief time. Third, you must not tolerate any interruptions during the Opening and Middle Conversations. Interruptions will be interpreted as an indication that you are distracted or in haste.

During the Middle Conversation you determine many important features of the present illness, outlined below. These features are the critical ones in bedside logic and it works best if you obtain them fully at the first opportunity, so you must not neglect or truncate the Middle Conversation. Most errors in bedside logic arise from neglect of the Middle Conversation.

In the Middle Conversation you ask specific questions that you need an answer to. Here, you begin to test your hypotheses about the disease process. You explore your ideas of the organ systems involved, the nature of the pathological process and the extent of that process. You generate questions to test your ideas as they develop: This is the essence of bedside logic.

It is important to avoid asking leading questions, those in which the form of the question implies an expected answer, since some patients tend to tell you what they think you want to hear. Your questions must be put in such a way that the patient understands that the possible responses, "yes," "no," and "sometimes" are all equally important. Thus a specific question about nausea accompanying an abdominal pain might be stated, "I need to know whether or not you ever get nauseated with your pain. Tell me if it ever occurs or never occurs or sometimes occurs." It works well to offer the patient choices to show that you have no preference for the response.

There is another problem with leading questions of the kind that are formed to indicate the expectation of a negative answer. When you ask, for example, "You never have nausea with your pain do you?" you may be misled by the answer. If nausea does not accompany the pain the usual native English-speaker will respond "No," meaning "No—I do not have nausea with the pain." The native Navajo-speaker (for example) will respond "Yes," meaning "Yes—I agree with you when you say that I do not have nausea with the pain." This problem may well exist as a linguistic variant in other languages. I have encountered it often when I, in a momentary lapse, have asked a leading question in this form.

The End Conversation

When you believe that you have exhausted the possibilities of the Middle Conversation you begin the End Conversation. This consists of a recitation by you of the story of the illness as you understand it so far. You repeat your understanding of the story of the illness, asking the patient to correct you when you are wrong. Give the patient the chance to add anything. Ask "Have I missed anything?" or "Is there anything I have said that is not quite correct?"

In this End Conversation not only are you trying to establish the complete story as you understand it, but also you are letting the patient know that you are beginning to formulate your ideas of what may be wrong. Your positions are temporarily reversed: He is listening and you are talking.

For this reason you must be careful to recognize the unexpressed fears and guilts of the patient, for in the End Conversation *he* is beginning to find out what *you* think. There are two important things to keep in mind in this connection.

First, patients who have complaints that they themselves do not understand often fear that they have a fatal illness, usually cancer.

Second, patients often conceal information from you that may be important, usually related to something that they are ashamed of like peculiar dietary practices, drug or substance abuse, sexual practices, and the like.

It is useful to introduce such matters at this time. If appropriate, it is helpful for you to say, for example, that the story suggests to you that the problem might be related to some drugs or medicines that the patient might be taking and that you want to know about them. If such sensitive matters are brought up by *you* in this End Conversation in a matter-of-fact way and you indicate why you are asking about them, most patients will respond freely. It is much better to get into such things in the End Conversation than to reserve them for the more interrogatory or confrontational setting of the routine questioning of the drug history. A point-blank question like "Do you ever shoot drugs?," without preparation, is an invitation to denial if the patient is sensitive about it.

In this way, the End Conversation can be used to lead into the other elements of the history that are usually organized as the drug history, the past history, the family history, the surgical history, and so on. It does not matter in what order these latter elements of the history are obtained. It is easiest if they are explored in whatever order seems natural.

In patients with gastrointestinal illness there is often a past history of several abdominal operations. Getting these straight in the Middle and End Conversations can sometimes be difficult. In such cases I have found it helpful to review abdominal operations later during the physical examination, when I can point to each scar and ask about the operation that led to it.

You should use the End Conversation to begin to bring the patient into your thinking process so far as you think that to be desirable at this point. Here you tell the patient, in effect, what other matters are important to you. This will lead naturally to a discussion of other matters that otherwise might seem to him to be unimportant.

The Rest of the History

The most important elements of the other parts of the history—the Past History, the Family History and so on—will have emerged in the three Conversations described above. You should, however, cover the routine elements that have not come up. This should be done after the End Conversation.

WHAT IS IMPORTANT TO THE PATIENT, AND WHY?

Patients want problems solved. You must learn what these problems are. The main problem is usually the major symptom. In general a patient will only volunteer to you what concerns him most. This may not be what most concerns you, but you must listen to what the patient says first, for this tells you both what he considers to be important and what most bothers him. This is the function of the Opening Conversation.

At some point you must discover why a particular aspect of the history concerns the patient most and you should not hesitate to ask why. "Why does this pain concern you so much?" or "Why do you worry so much about this pain?" are questions that often yield answers which illustrate the magnitude of the problem or reveal specific fears or hitherto-concealed elements of the history. I often ask "What do you think is causing your problem?" This question often brings out previously unexpressed fears and sometimes give you an unsuspected lead to correct understanding.

WHAT IS IMPORTANT TO YOU?

Patients rarely appreciate what is important to you. You uncover this in the Middle Conversation.

In talking with patients you should pay attention not only to the answers to your questions but also to specific nonverbal communications. The meanings of some behavioral responses—weeping, hostile words, and the like—are obvious. Others are more subtle: blushing, hesitancy in response, stammering, even a particular choice of words in response to a question may warn you that you have touched a tender spot. By constantly watching the patient, you may pick up many important clues in "body language" like shifting in position, clenching of the fists, partial covering of the face with the hand, crossing or uncrossing of the legs, rubbing the hands, clutching at the chest or abdomen, glancing at an accompanying relative, smoothing the hair, and so on. Such actions may suggest anger, shame, fear, or depression (Tables 1-1 to 1-4). It is usually best, when you detect such signals, to pursue the matter at once. You should indicate that you sense a particular concern about a matter that prompts such a response. You should ask about such concerns. Say "You look like you are about to cry," or "You seem to be angry—tell me about how you are feeling." Such inquiry may prompt tears or a tirade in a patient who is suppressing strong feelings. You will often learn about important things that he has not told you about from such exchanges.

Be cautious in how you interpret evidence of extreme emotional responses a patient may show to his illness or to your conversation. Extreme responses suggest emotional instability or neuroticism and it is easy for you to leap to the conclusion that the symptoms are a consequence of such emotional instability. But people react to illness in many ways and emotionally labile people may show far stronger reactions to illness than you are accustomed to seeing. The idea that a symptom is the consequence of neuroticism is easy to get but hard to prove. The rule I follow is always to give the patient the benefit of the doubt. I always assume that I am dealing with a complaint of organic origin. When a patient tells you that his complaint is aggravated in situations that produce anxiety or stress, do not assume therefore that anxiety is the sole source of the illness. Many symptoms of organic origin, like angina pectoris, are made worse by anxiety. Conversely many symptoms regress when patients are distracted or preoccupied by something else. It is not rare for soldiers injured in battle or

Table 1-1. Some Signs that Mainly Indicate Anger or Resentment

Clenching the jaws
Clenching the fists
Uncrossing the legs and sitting upright
Gripping the table or chair
Smoking or asking to smoke
Glancing angrily at a relative

Table 1-2. Some Signs that Mainly Indicate Embarrassment

Leaning back and crossing the legs and/or arms
Rubbing the palms of the hands together
Partially covering the jaw or mouth with the hand
Smoothing the hair
Breaking eye contact with you
Glancing fearfully at a relative

Table 1-3. Some Signs that Mainly Indicate Fear

Constant and intense eye contact
Sweating and/or pallor
Clutching or rubbing a piece of clothing, a handkerchief, a piece of tissue or a purse
Shifting the chair away from you
Inappropriate laughter, giggling or smiling
Abnormally rapid or deep breathing

Table 1-4. Some Signs that Mainly Indicate Depression

An expressionless face
Paucity of body movements
Avoidance of eye contact
A slumping posture
Difficulty in following the line of conversation
Poor grooming

athletes injured on the playing-field to discover the injury only later when the distraction is gone.

Later chapters of this book deal with the major complaints or principal symptoms that apply to gastrointestinal disease. These are *trouble in swallowing, heartburn, pain in the abdomen, diarrhea, constipation, incontinence of stool, painful defecation, jaundice, blood in the stool, nausea and vomiting,* and *gas and bloating.* There are six specific features of these complaints that you should explore during the Middle Conversation: *character* (including *severity*), *location, chronology, aggravating factors, relieving factors,* and *associated symptoms.* You should examine these general features of the major complaints in all cases. I always make a conscious and deliberate effort to cover these matters in each patient in order not to miss anything.

SOME SPECIFIC FEATURES OF COMPLAINTS THAT YOU MUST COVER

Character

A patient may denote the principal symptom with a term that says little about the actual character of the symptom. For example, a patient with abdominal pain rarely describes the nature of the pain without direct inquiry. In the case of a complaint that is an abnormal sensation, the question should be very general at first, "What does it feel like?" It is particularly helpful to offer lay terms to allow the patient to choose words that he feels accurately describe the sensation. You should also ask how a symptom affects work, sleep, eating, or other activities. In this way you can judge the severity of the problem. I find it hard to judge severity by asking directly—severity is a very subjective matter and the perception of severity varies a great deal among people.

Location

The feature of location obviously does not have much relevance to a principal complaint like blood in the stool, diarrhea, and constipation, but it does apply to the sensory complaints. When a patient is asked for the location of an abnormal sensation, he will usually put his hand in the area. You should make him indicate as precisely as possible where the sensation seems to be centered, where it is less intense, and where it seems to radiate. Ask him to point with one finger. Location is especially important in interpreting the organ of origin of abdominal pain.

Chronology

A precise chronology of a symptom or set of symptoms is always critical in the interpretation of symptoms. A patient almost never tells you all that you need to know about chronology, and so you must make a special effort to understand the chronology of an illness.

Chronology includes several elements: nature of onset, rate of progression, and duration and intervals of attacks and remissions. When you ask about the date of the onset of a complaint you will usually get a quite specific response for an illness that started recently, but a very vague answer for an event of remote or insidious onset. When a patient is vague you can make use of special events—seasonal changes, secular or religious holidays, major historical and political events, or birthdays—to try to establish time of onset. Chronology is also important in relation to aggravating and relieving factors. With abdominal pain that is aggravated by eating, for example, the rapidity of the effect is often useful to know.

Aggravating Factors

Many of the principal complaints in gastroenterology are made worse by certain normal gastrointestinal events like eating and defecation, or by nongastrointestinal events like posture, activity, deep breathing, and the use of medications. Such aggravating factors are often quite suggestive of certain causes of symptoms and you must ask about them in detail.

Relieving Factors

Most patients with one of the principal complaints will have tried one or another of the common maneuvers known to laymen that are used to obtain relief. This information is often not volunteered. A patient usually volunteers statements about what makes a symptom worse, but he less commonly tells you what makes a symptom better. Like aggravating factors, relieving factors are often very specific for the origins of complaints. They may be related to normal gastrointestinal functions like eating and defecation, or to nongastrointestinal events like posture, activity, and the use of medications. It is important for you to know not only what induces relief, but also what things have been tried that fail to produce relief.

Related Symptoms

The chapters that follow deal with a set of symptoms that are usually the major symptoms in gastroenterology. Of course, they may occur together or they may be associated with other relatively minor symptoms. If the principal symptom is severe a patient often neglects to mention related symptoms. These related symptoms are very useful in your interpretation of a history and you must always ask about them. There may be many that are not overtly gastrointestinal—sweating, dizziness, pounding of the heart, headache, weakness, and so on. The absence of related symptoms is just as important as their presence.

THE CHOICE OF TERMS IN TALKING WITH PATIENTS

The vocabularies of physicians and the vocabularies of patients are quite different. Vocabularies are culturally determined. Highly educated patients use different terms than do uneducated patients. Patients with a native language that is not English may use different English terms from those used by native English-speakers. Even in the native English-speaking world, different terms are used for the same thing from one geographic region to another. You must be aware of these things if you are to understand exactly what you are hearing. You must be sure that you know what a patient is actually saying.

In gastroenterology the conversation often deals with matters that may be considered in some circles to be vulgar. These things must be talked about, but a patient may find it difficult to speak of them because he hesitates to use terms that he considers to be crude. This presents a special problem in gastroenterology, for you must use terms that the patient can understand, but you must not use vulgar terms yourself.

You can best solve this problem by interrupting the patient to offer terms or definitions of terms that he may find useful to explain his problem. Thus, a patient may say "I have the shits," or, from the other end of the spectrum, "I have difficulty controlling my bowels." Since both expressions are not precise you should interrupt at once to say "What do you mean by that? Tell me exactly how you have difficulty with your stools." This problem in language is explored further in subsequent chapters dealing with specific complaints, but the following general principles apply in all cases.

First, be prepared to hear anything from the most vulgar to the most refined terms.

Second, be sure that you understand at once, in the plainest possible language, what the patient means by the terms that he uses. Offer him terms or phrases, if necessary, that are simple, straightforward, and clear.

Third, do not yourself use terms that the patient may consider to be vulgar. Maintain professionalism in your own language.

WHEN TO WRITE THINGS DOWN

I stated before that you should not take notes while you are eliciting the story of the illness because it impedes the natural flow of the conversation. In the subsequent steps of history-taking, reviewing the past history, family history and so on, it is natural to take notes, for this part of the process assumes more the character of an interview than a conversation. Explain to the patient that you must take notes because you might have trouble remembering some relatively minor points. Also, this part of the history involves the assembly of facts that are not so clearly related to the illness, so notes are helpful. After the history-taking process is complete you can write the whole account from memory for the current illness and from your notes for the rest.

THE SYNTHESIS OF A LOGICAL STORY

A patient never volunteers all the information that you want to know, or should want to know, in order for you to put together a logical story. This is true mostly because a patient does not know or recognize what is important and partly because he may not volunteer something out of feelings of fear or guilt. The assembly of a coherent and logical story requires you to exercise the faculty of synthesis, the ability to assemble a set of observations (some made by the patient and others made by you), to place these in relation to one another, to estimate their relative proportions, and to make of them something that is more than the sum of the parts.

Of course you must allow the patient to tell his complete story as he sees it at the outset. This is the function of the Opening Conversation. You fill in the details of the story in the Middle Conversation. It is here that you exert the synthetic force to create a story that is logical and complete from the mixed-up and incomplete story of the Opening Conversation. The process of synthesis lies in identifying the neglected elements of the story and fitting all the elements together to see what the story implies in physiologic terms. This synthetic process has two elements, one of organization and one of interpretation. Organization and interpretation occur simultaneously and are mutually reinforcing processes in your mind. For example, when a patient says that he has trouble swallowing, he will rarely volunteer those specific foods that cause the trouble. Certain causes of trouble in swallowing quite specifically produce symptoms only with the swallowing of certain foods, information that can be very useful in differential diagnosis. You must know this and usually you must ask about it—thus you are interpreting and organizing the clinical information simultaneously.

Patients often have two or more gastrointestinal complaints or problems that seem to be separate or only remotely related. In that case you should describe and analyze them as separate problems. When a patient presents two major complaints that may be related, like two kinds of abdominal pain, you should try at the outset to see if they are related or separable. I ask the patient directly for his opinion about this and his reasons for his opinion.

THE SUMMARY CONVERSATION

After the history and the subsequent physical examination are completed, you should have a quite complete list of ideas in mind as to the nature of the problem. That is, you should have compiled a list of the disordered physiologic processes that could account for the symptoms. This should be a list of general pathologic processes like inflammatory disease of the stomach or a bleeding site in the colon, rather than established nosologic entities like gastric ulcer or colonic carcinoma. It is important that you keep your ideas in the form of pathologic processes rather than "diseases" at this point because you will avoid the pitfall of arriving at a diagnosis prematurely, before all the evidence is in.

After you have completed the whole bedside examination, the complete history and the physical examination, it is both courteous and useful for you to give the patient a brief summary of your thinking. Patients who have complaints that they do not understand usually fear that they have cancer or some other mortal condition. You need not mention cancer in this Summary Conversation, even if you suspect it, but if you think that the condition is as serious as that you can convey this by your demeanor and choice of language. On the contrary, if the condition appears to be less ominous, like an inflammation, you can similarly convey that idea indirectly. You should tell the patient, in terms that he can understand, the general nature of the problem that you suspect to be present, avoiding terms for specific nosologic entities. For example, if you suspect one of the inflammatory bowel diseases, to name them at this point is to invite questions about the cause, treatment, prognosis, and the like. It is nonproductive to do that at this time. It raises fears, introduces confusion, and wastes time. It is better to say only that you suspect an inflammation of the bowel, that there are many forms of such inflammation and that further tests should reveal which one may be present. A patient may press you for a specific diagnosis and prognosis during this Summary Conversation. I tell him that I will discuss such specifics later when all the necessary information is at hand. When you promise to do that be sure that you follow through.

At this point in the conversation you should explain the further tests that you propose to do, why you will do them, in what order you will do them, and what information will be gained. Patients should always know what they are in for and they should know you are aware of the discomfort that may occur in this testing. A little time spent in explaining the planned tests usually reduces anxiety and delay when the tests are done.

A SUMMARY OF THE MAIN POINTS OF THIS CHAPTER

I. Preparatory Strategies
   A. Purposes
      1. To establish the setting for a formal conversation.
      2. To establish your position, as physician, as the leader of the conversation.
      3. To make sure that the conversation will be private, relaxed, and complete.
   B. Methods
      1. Arrange the room so that you and the patient are seated 3 to 6 feet apart without an intervening desk or table, with your faces slightly oblique to one another.
      2. Allow other people to be present only at the request of or with the permission of the patient.
      3. Establish your leadership position in the conversation by introducing yourself and observing the usual formalities of beginning a conversation.

II. The Opening Conversation
   A. Purposes
      1. To establish the general features of the illness as the patient knows them.
      2. To find out what the patient considers to be most important to *him*.

B. Methods
1. Invite the patient to tell his story, indicating what you may already know of the nature of the illness.
2. Let the patient talk until he seems to have completed the story.
3. If the patient seems to ramble get him back on course gently.
4. Do not take notes.
5. Maintain eye contact.
6. Allow no interruptions.
7. Watch for clues to unexpressed anger, embarrassment, fear, and depression in the patient's facial expression, word choice, and body language.

III. The Middle Conversation
A. Purposes
1. To fill in details of the illness that the patient has neglected to mention.
2. To find out points that are important to *you*.

B. Methods
1. Ask questions about the character, location, chronology, aggravating factors, relieving factors, and associated symptoms, as necessary, for the main and secondary features of the illness.
2. Do not ask leading questions.
3. Do not take notes.
4. Maintain eye contact.
5. Allow no interruptions.
6. Watch for clues to unexpressed anger, embarrassment, fear, or depression in the patient's facial expression, word choice, and body language.
7. Explore any suspected anger, embarrassment, fear, or depression that you detect.
8. Be sure that you know exactly what the patient is saying by being sure that you both understand the terms that you both use.
9. As you fill in the details of the illness, organize and interpret what you are learning in order to synthesize a story that makes sense on physiologic grounds.

IV. The End Conversation
A. Purposes
1. To review the story of the illness as you understand it in order to verify all details.
2. To let the patient know that you are beginning to formulate a list of physiologically defined diagnostic possibilities.
3. To lead naturally into the other elements of the history—the drug history, surgical history, past history, and the like.

B. Methods
1. Tell the story as you understand it, asking the patient to interrupt to correct you if you are wrong and to complete any details.
2. Suggest briefly what you consider to be the general nature of the physiologic basis for the illness, to the extent that seems desirable.

V. The Summary Conversation (after completion of the rest of the history and the physical examination)

A. Purposes
   1. To summarize your thoughts about the diagnostic possibilities in physiologic terms so that the patient knows at least something of what you suspect.
   2. To indicate to the patient what you want to do in further diagnostic testing and what those tests will involve.
B. Methods
   1. Explain your thinking in terms the patient will understand.
   2. Do not bring up specific nosologic entities—speak only in terms of physiologic processes.
   3. Show that you understand the difficulties of further testing and explain the reasons for further testing.

2

TROUBLE WITH SWALLOWING, AND HEARTBURN

INTRODUCTION

The organs involved in swallowing have three functions: the transport of things that are swallowed from the mouth to the stomach, the opposition to reflux of gastric contents into the esophagus, and the clearance from the esophagus of any gastric contents that do reflux into the esophagus.

Motions of the walls of the pharynx and esophagus accomplish these functions. The analysis of symptoms of disordered structure and function of the swallowing apparatus can quite precisely indicate the nature of the lesion. This chapter outlines the relevant structures and functions, characterizes the symptoms of dysfunction, discusses the ways in which the symptoms arise and presents specific examples of clinical entities that produce these symptoms.

The symptoms of difficulty in the swallowing process are difficult swallowing (dysphagia), painful swallowing (odynophagia), and heartburn (pyrosis). The idea that a symptom called globus hystericus or the globus sensation is a swallowing disorder has somehow gotten into the minds of many people. It certainly is not. The globus sensation is the feeling of a lump in the throat that *does not* interfere with swallowing. This is a common sensation associated with feelings of grief; a somewhat similar sensation sometimes occurs with heartburn. The important point is that the symptoms of trouble with swallowing and heartburn *never* arise from emotional disturbances. You can nearly always find an organic explanation in patients with heartburn and with trouble in swallowing if you know what to ask about and what to look for.

THE RELEVANT ANATOMY AND ORGAN PHYSIOLOGY

The Anatomy

The muscular walls of the pharynx and esophagus have distinctive subdivisions, but they work together. You should consider the entire system as a tubular conduit containing a series of connected elements that are anatomically and functionally distinct, yet functionally integrated.

The pharynx is the fusiform organ behind the mouth that connects to the mouth and nose and to the trachea and esophagus. The muscular walls of the pharynx constitute three overlapping sheets of striated muscle, the pharyngeal constrictors. The most caudad part of the inferior pharyngeal constrictor is thickened to form a distinct muscle band, the cricopharyngeus muscle (Fig. 2-1). This striated muscle, which is the upper esophageal sphincter, joins the ends of the cricoid cartilage. Its contraction compresses the esophageal lumen against the arc of the cricoid cartilage to close the opening to the esophagus by forming a transverse slit. The body of the esophagus begins at the lower edge of the cricopharyngeus muscle and contains two layers of muscle, the outer longitudinal and the inner circular. This is striated muscle in both layers to a point about one-third of the way down the esophagus, 7 cm below the pharyngoesophageal junction. Here, striated muscle is replaced by smooth muscle, the two types of muscle interdigitating over several centimeters. Just above the stomach the circular layer of smooth muscle is thickened for a few centimeters at the level where the squamous epithelium (which lines the pharynx and esophagus) joins the glandular epithelium of the stomach at an irregular margin called the Z-line. This muscular thickening is the lower esophageal sphincter; it normally lies at or just above the level of the hiatus in the diaphragm through which the esophagus passes (Fig. 2-2).

The ninth and tenth cranial nerves innervate the whole segment involved in swallowing, the ninth nerve innervating the pharynx and the tenth nerve supplying the upper esophageal sphincter and the rest of the esophagus.

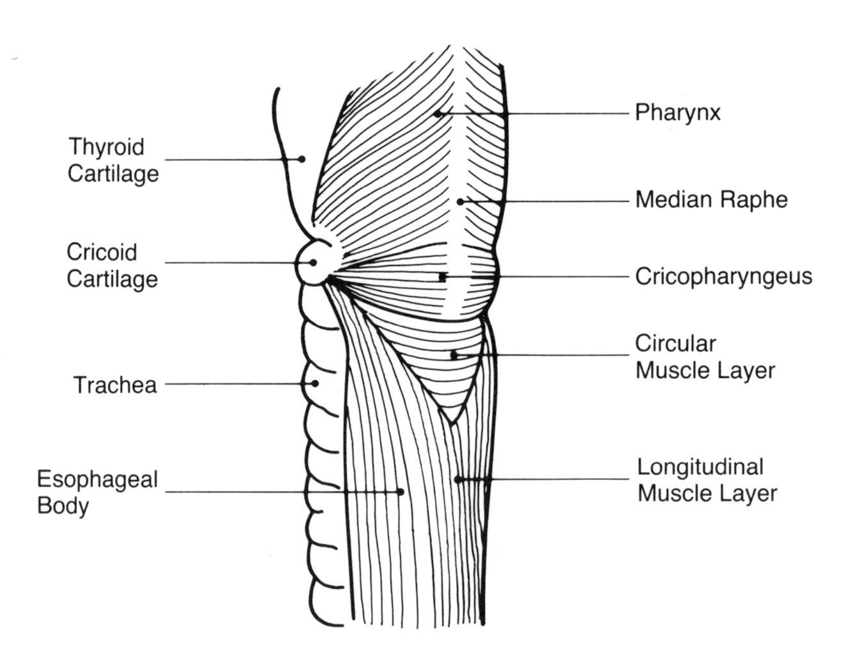

Fig. 2-1. A posterior oblique view of the cephalic end of the esophagus to show the arrangements of the musculature.

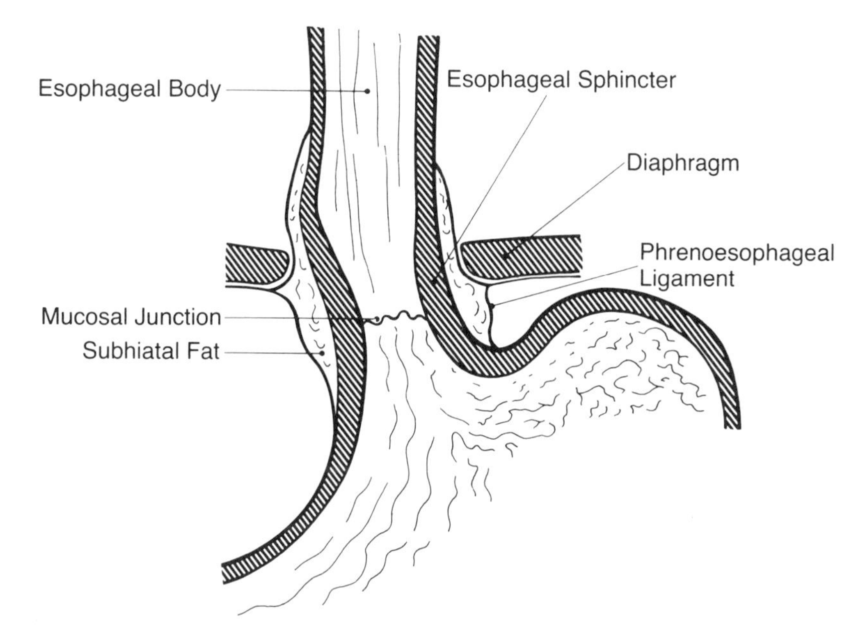

Fig. 2-2. A saggital section of the caudal end of the esophagus to show its structure and its relation to adjacent structures.

Functions and Control of Functions

In considering function you must think of five segments: the pharynx, the upper esophageal sphincter, the striated-muscle esophageal body, the smooth-muscle esophageal body, and the lower esophageal sphincter.

The Pharynx

The pharynx is nearly flaccid at rest, though the striated muscle exhibits a variable degree of tone. In swallowing, a series of rapid movements occurs in the mouth and pharynx in a patterned sequence. The tongue is elevated to force the bolus into the oropharynx and the soft palate rises to seal off the nasopharynx from the oropharynx. The pharyngeal constrictors contract peristaltically as a unit so that the advancing face of the contraction moves caudad as a front to force the bolus toward the esophagus. The parapharyngeal muscles elevate and displace the pharynx and larynx to direct the bolus toward the esophagus. The epiglottis is moved over the laryngeal inlet. These motions are all brought about by excitation of the striated muscle by nerves that are like the somatic nerves that innervate somatic striated muscle; there are no intermediate synapses like those in autonomic nerve pathways and the nerves contact the striated muscle through endplates where the transmitter is acetylcholine and the receptor is nicotinic. These nerves originate in motor nuclei in the brainstem and traverse the ninth cranial nerves.

The Upper Esophageal Sphincter

The upper esophageal sphincter is strongly and tonically contracted at rest to seal the esophageal lumen. In swallowing, this tonic contraction disappears for less than a second to allow the bolus to enter the esophagus. Relaxation of this contracted sphincter begins during pharyngeal peristalsis and it ends as pharyngeal peristalsis ends. The tonic contraction at rest is a consequence of a tonic activity of the somatic motor nerves that excite contraction of the striated muscle. The relaxation in a swallow is a result of transient suppression of this tonic nerve activity. These nerves originate in motor nuclei in the brainstem and traverse the tenth cranial nerves.

The Striated-Muscle Part of the Esophageal Body

The striated-muscle part of the esophageal body is flaccid at rest. The upper esophageal sphincter contracts after its transient relaxation in swallowing and a contraction simultaneously begins in the circular muscle layer of the esophageal body at the most cephalad level. This contraction moves as a front through the circular layer of striated muscle toward the stomach. The contraction represents the transient excitation of the striated muscle by its somatic innervation. The contraction is peristaltic because motor units, groups of striated muscle cells sharing a single common motor nerve, are excited in a craniocaudad sequence.

The Smooth-Muscle Part of the Esophageal Body

The smooth-muscle part of the esophageal body is also flaccid at rest. After a swallow it generates a caudally directed peristaltic ring of contraction, the contraction appearing to be a continuation of the peristaltic contraction of the striated-muscle part of the esophageal body. This contraction arises from excitation of the circular layer of smooth muscle by autonomic nerves. Autonomic fibers that originate in the brainstem and traverse the tenth cranial nerve excite secondary nerves in the myenteric plexus of the smooth-muscled part of the esophageal body. These secondary motor nerves excite the muscle to contract. The contraction is peristaltic because of gradients in the smooth muscle along the esophageal body and because of a craniocaudad sequence in the activation of the nerves of the myenteric plexus. The neurohumoral transmitter of the responsible motor nerves is unknown.

The Lower Esophageal Sphincter

The lower esophageal sphincter is tonically contracted at rest to seal the lumen in a rosette at the esophagogastric junction. This tonic contraction is mostly myogenic, due to special properties of this smooth muscle, but it is modified by excitatory and inhibitory nerves. The smooth muscle of the sphincter relaxes in swallowing, the relaxation beginning at about the time peristalsis in the esophageal body begins and ending when peristalsis is completed. The relaxation is the result of activation of autonomic fibers in the tenth cranial nerve which act on secondary nerve cells in the myenteric plexus that inhibit the muscle by release of an unknown neurohumoral transmitter.

Integration of Pharyngeal and Esophageal Movements

The functions of the five distinguishable elements of the swallowing apparatus are closely coordinated and their integration is constant, so these movements show very little variation in their timing from one swallow to another. This is true largely because the activation of the elements occurs by way of extrinsic nerves, all arising from nerve cells that lie close together in the brainstem in the floor of the fourth ventricle. These cells make up the motor nuclei of the ninth and tenth cranial nerves (Fig. 2-3). The swallowing center, adjacent to these nuclei, coordinates their discharge (Fig. 2-4). The swallowing center is programmed to discharge by volition. Its activation is facilitated by certain sensory inputs, including those produced by closure of the jaw and elevation of the tongue. In discharging, the swallowing center interacts with the somatic motor nerve cells in the cranial nerve nuclei in a fixed order, exciting some motor units in a craniocaudad sequence to produce peristalsis in striated muscle of the pharynx and proximal esophagus, and inhibiting others to relax the striated muscle of the upper esophageal sphincter. The center also activates the autonomic motor nerve cells in the cranial nerve nuclei that excite peristalsis in the smooth muscle of the distal esophageal body and relax the lower esophageal sphincter. In the smooth-muscled segments (the distal esophageal body and the lower esophageal sphincter) local circuits in the myenteric plexus can also maintain full coordination of function. Localized distension of the distal esophagus produces esophageal peristalsis in this region and relaxation of the sphincter.

Flow in the Pharyngoesophageal Conduit

In a swallow, the tongue presses the bolus into the pharynx. Pharyngeal peristalsis carries the bolus toward the esophagus, this flow being facilitated by the shift in pharyngeal position brought about by the contractions of the parapharyngeal muscles. The relaxation of the upper sphincter allows the bolus to enter the esophagus with essentially no delay. Because the esophageal body is flaccid and empty and since we eat in an erect posture, a very liquid bolus passes through the esophageal body largely by gravity alone so that some fluid may reach the lower esophageal sphincter before full sphincteric relaxation has occurred. In this case peristalsis clears the esophageal body of that part of the liquid bolus that has remained coating the esophageal mucosa. Boluses that are larger, more solid, or more viscous are less likely to fall through the esophagus by gravity because of the frictional resistance offered by the mucosa. The saliva which accompanies the swallowed bolus lubricates the bolus to reduce this frictional resistance. Such large, solid, or viscous boluses move largely because

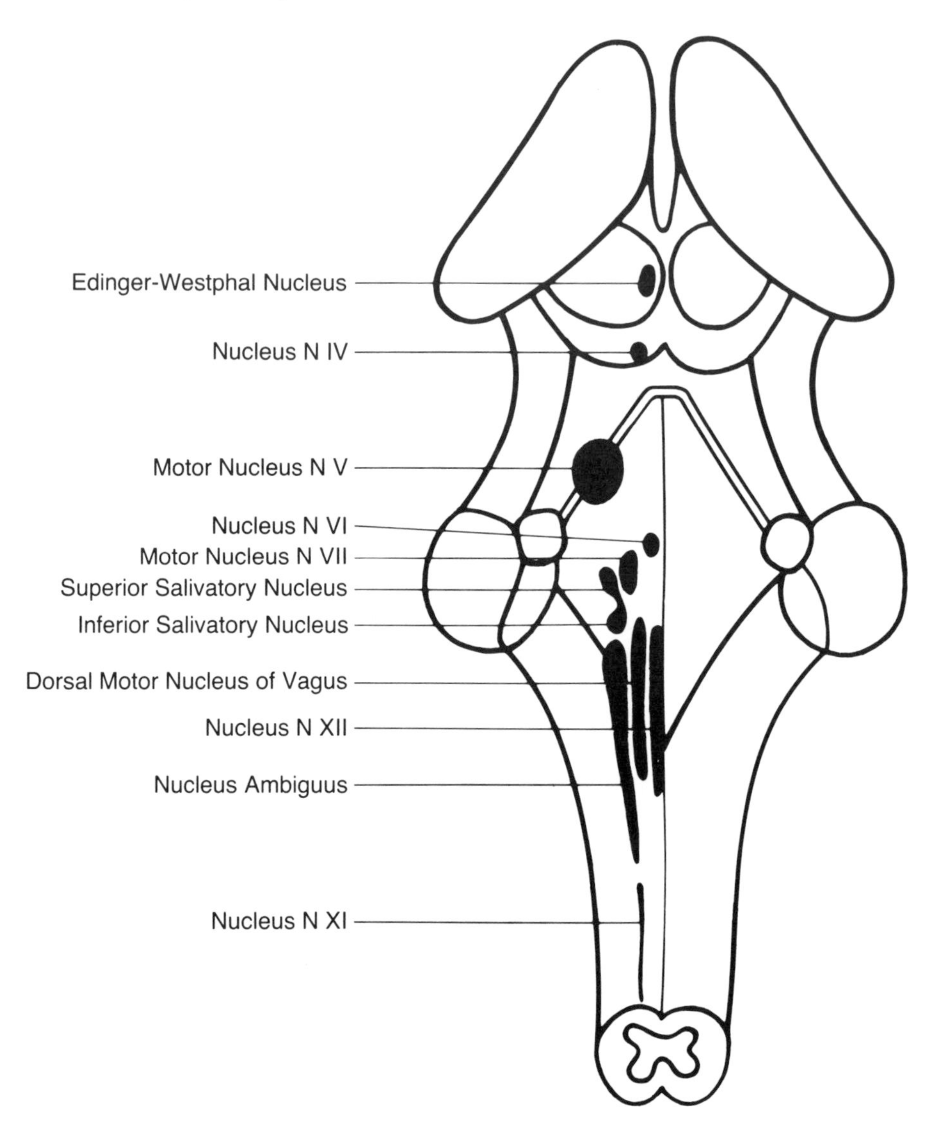

Fig. 2-3. The motor nuclei of the region of the fourth ventricle. They are drawn only on one side. Note that the two vagal motor nuclei, the dorsal motor nucleus and the nucleus ambiguus, are very close together and that they lie close to the nuclei of the adjacent cranial nerves.

they are pushed by the peristaltic wave. Whatever the character of the bolus, the lower esophageal sphincter relaxes early enough in the swallowing sequence that there is only a momentary slowing of progress of the bolus into the stomach.

Variable quantities of gastric content normally reflux into the esophagus from time to time, more so when the stomach is filled and when the person is recumbent. These episodes of gastroesophageal reflux occur because of brief spontaneous relaxations of the lower esophageal sphincter. The refluxed bolus,

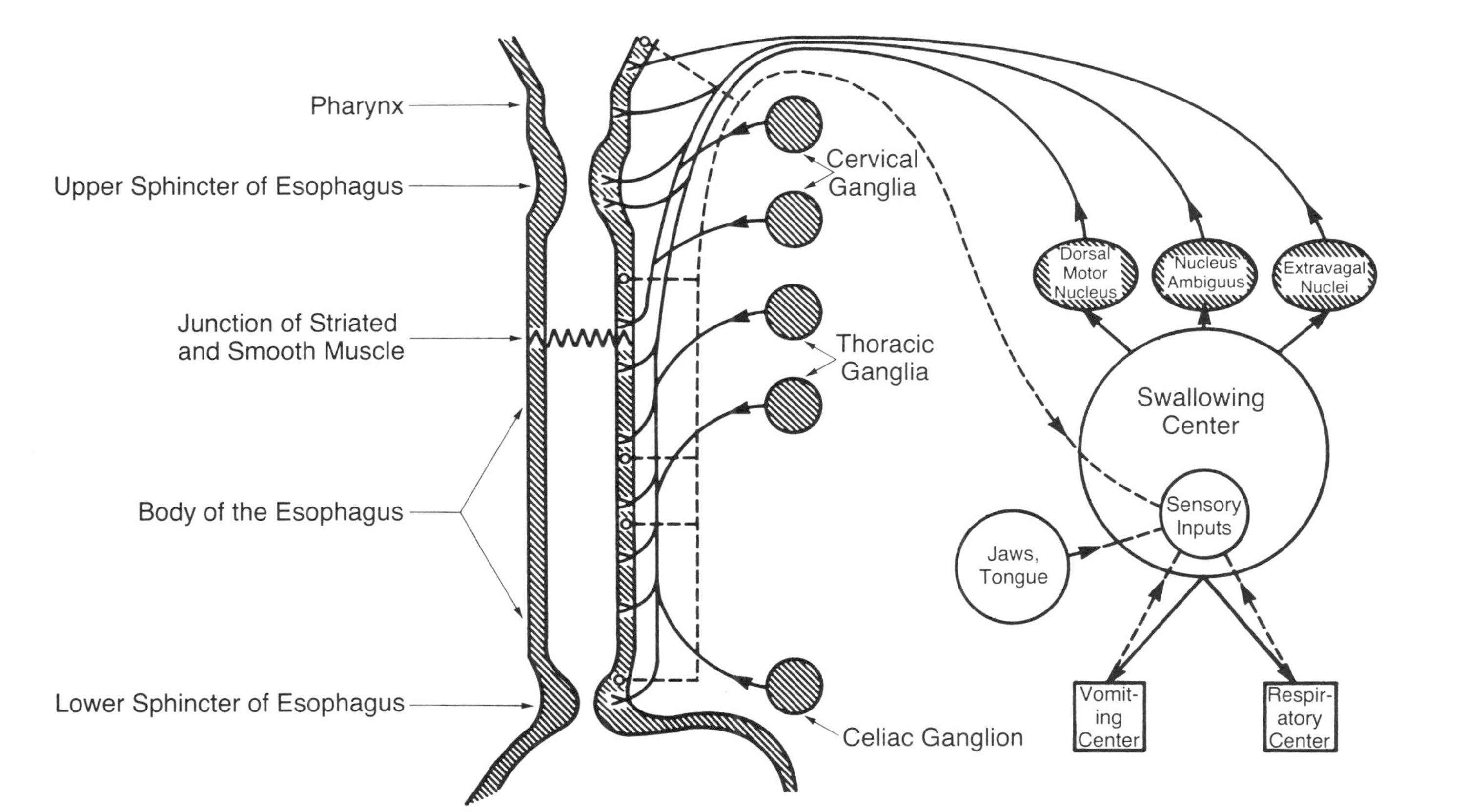

Fig. 2-4. The extramural nerves that supply the esophagus. Motor pathways are drawn as solid lines while sensory pathways are shown as dashed lines. The central nerve centers are at the right, the esophagus at the left. (Adapted from Christensen J: The esophagus. p. 75. In Christensen J, Wingate DL (eds): A Guide to Gastrointestinal Mobility. John Wright, PSG, Bristol, England, 1983.)

either by distending the esophagus or by exciting mucosal chemoreceptors, stimulates local circuits in the myenteric plexus to establish reflex peristalsis in the smooth-muscled segment. Such local reflex peristalsis is called secondary peristalsis to distinguish it from primary peristalsis, which is initiated by a swallow. Thus refluxed boluses are quickly cleared from the distal esophagus.

DIFFICULTY IN SWALLOWING—DYSPHAGIA

The Origins of Dysphagia

Dysphagia arises from any lesion or malfunction that impairs the flow of a swallowed bolus along the pharyngoesophageal conduit. Dysphagia always means that the freedom of the lumen to receive the bolus is restricted in some way. Increased resistance to bolus movement most commonly arises within the conduit itself, for the motive forces that propel the bolus also arise within the passageway. Dysphagia is not often caused by displacement of the conduit by an extraluminal mass, for displacement of the whole organ displaces both the lumen and the motor apparatus. Extrinsic lesions produce dysphagia when they encircle the conduit to narrow the lumen by concentric compression, when they become attached to the passageway to interfere with wall motion in contraction, or when they compress the conduit against the spine.

The Specific Features of Dysphagia

The Character of Dysphagia

When a patient says he senses some difficulty in swallowing, or that "food sticks," he is describing dysphagia. Dysphagia means simply a sense of difficulty in the process of swallowing. Normal people are almost unaware of the complex motions and the flows that occur in swallowing. You are aware of the jaw and tongue movements and of part of the pharyngeal contraction but you sense nothing beyond that point. At its mildest, dysphagia is only the awareness of some sensation that follows pharyngeal contraction. More severe dysphagia is a sense of transient slowing of the passage of a bolus. At worst it is a sense of obstruction, a feeling that the bolus has lodged at some point. In true dysphagia these feelings do not seem to be really painful.

There are two kinds of dysphagia: oropharyngeal and esophageal. These are distinguishable on the basis of certain specific features of the complaint. They signify different classes of disorders, so you must distinguish between them. Oropharyngeal dysphagia represents disordered function of the pharynx; esophageal dysphagia reflects disordered esophageal function.

The Location of Dysphagia

A patient usually attempts to show you where he perceives the sensation of dysphagia (Fig. 2-5). If he does not, ask him to do so. The location of this sensation above the suprasternal notch suggests oropharyngeal dysphagia. Pha-

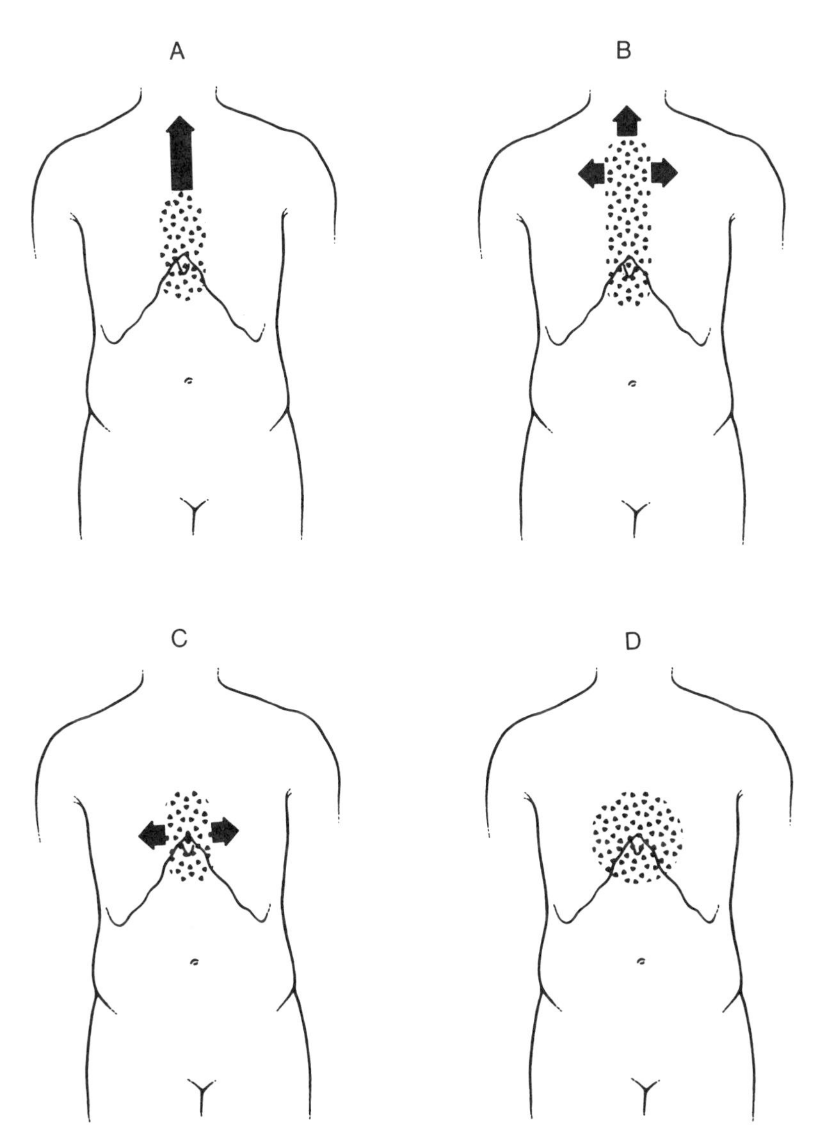

Fig. 2-5. Some common patterns of distribution of esophageal sensations including pain. These patterns apply both to mucosal and muscular pains. **(A)** The most common pattern, in which pain radiates from the primary location (shaded area) toward the neck (arrow). **(B & C)** These patterns are easily confused with those of cardiac pain because of the lateral radiation. Such radiation is sometimes unilateral. **(D)** The pattern in Figure D is common for the heartburn of distal chronic esophagitis.

ryngeal sensation is quite accurately perceived at this level, anteriorly in the throat. When the location is at or below the suprasternal notch the source of dysphagia is most likely to be in the esophagus. In esophageal dysphagia the precise location of the sensation in the chest does not indicate the level of the lesion. Usually the location is perceived more proximally than the lesion, and quite widely. The sensation commonly occurs in the anterior chest, infrequently in the back, and almost never in the epigastrium.

The Chronology of Dysphagia

Patients commonly cannot date the onset of esophageal dysphagia, probably because many normal people have an occasional episode. Also, with many causes, the dysphagia is so mild or intermittent at first that it is ignored. A patient rarely seeks medical attention when he has had only one episode unless it is an episode of complete esophageal obstruction. Patients usually date the onset of oropharyngeal dysphagia more accurately, probably because oropharyngeal dysphagia is not a part of normal experience. Patients recognize it immediately as something abnormal. You should ask about the acuteness of the onset for it may help you to distinguish oropharyngeal dysphagia from esophageal dysphagia when the sensation is at the suprasternal notch and the other features of the symptoms do not help you much to make the distinction.

You must explore the progression of dysphagia. When dysphagia progresses steadily from intermittent episodes with solids to more frequent episodes with liquid boluses, you must suspect a cancer. With stable causes of dysphagia the episodes are commonly intermittent and occur only with rather solid boluses, at least for a long time. The rate of progression is important. In cancer the dysphagia progresses to become severe over a few months; the benign causes may not lead to severe dysphagia for a year or more. These more stable benign causes include inflammatory strictures, mucosal webs, and rings. Even in the motor disorders of the esophagus, which are fairly constant once they have developed, progression is slow and the dysphagia characteristically remains intermittent for a long time. In the nonmalignant causes the dysphagia commonly remains intermittent because abnormalities in the pharyngoesophageal conduit (both abnormal motor processes and obstructions) are not the only factors that can impair bolus progression. The lubricating action of the saliva, the size of the swallowed bolus, and the degree of chewing are all important as well. For this reason episodes of dysphagia may occur only in relation to certain circumstances, when patients are not chewing well. This occurs when they are eating rapidly, eating in a social situation where they are talking to other people, or after a sudden change in the teeth. The small volume of saliva swallowed with boluses in rapid eating and the reduced volume secreted in scleroderma and in aging are sometimes important factors in dysphagia.

In oropharyngeal dysphagia, you may see a very sudden onset with a trend to slow improvement. This pattern strongly suggests an extrinsic neuropathic lesion, usually a brainstem stroke.

Aggravating Factors in Dysphagia

Patients with oropharyngeal dysphagia usually have trouble with almost anything they eat or drink. Liquids usually cause more trouble than solids because they flow more easily into the trachea or nasopharynx.

Patients with esophageal dysphagia frequently note that the dysphagia is worse with solids than with liquids, or that it occurs more in some circumstances than in others. Solids that are commonly not chewed well are usually the most troublesome; these include meat (especially "dry" meat) and peanut butter. Sometimes drinking very cold liquids or eating ice cream will make dysphagia worse. This is very suggestive of esophageal spasm, but it is not invariably present. Dysphagia is often noticed by patients to occur mainly at banquets, family dinners, or business lunches. This may only mean that patients do not chew thoroughly on such occasions, that the symptom is worsened by anxiety, or that they best recall those episodes that precipitated embarrassment.

Relieving Factors in Dysphagia

A patient with esophageal dysphagia usually tries to relieve dysphagia only when the feeling lasts for some time. He usually tries drinking something (to "wash it down"). If this gives no relief he may try to induce vomiting. Relief by such maneuvers has little diagnostic significance. It only means that a bolus has lodged for some time. Patients rarely seek or find any other way to relieve esophageal dysphagia, for example, by the use of medications. Most patients recognize the aggravating factors and seek to avoid them. Patients with oropharyngeal dysphagia commonly find some relief if they chew carefully, eat slowly, and swallow cautiously.

Associated Symptoms in Dysphagia

When dysphagia is perceived in the anterior neck you must ask if swallowed liquids ever come up into the nose, or if the patient ever chokes or coughs on swallowing. Such nasopharyngeal reflux or aspiration of swallowed liquids signifies dysfunction of the pharyngeal motor apparatus and identifies oropharyngeal dysphagia.

Weight loss is obviously often related to dysphagia. You must ask about weight loss because that gives you an estimate of the severity of the problem. Most people with dysphagia try hard to maintain nutrition by altering the diet or the pattern of eating, and they are often quite successful in doing so even when the dysphagia is severe or prolonged. Significant weight loss strongly suggests a constant and major cause, like a malignant obstruction, a very narrow stricture, or a very severe motor abnormality.

PAINFUL SWALLOWING—ODYNOPHAGIA

The Origins of Odynophagia

The pain of odynophagia may arise either from the mucosa or from the muscular wall. The nerves that mediate the pain must be different in some way from those that mediate the sensation of dysphagia, for dysphagia may progress to its most severe state without becoming painful, while patients with odynophagia that fades as the causative lesion regresses do not usually pass through a phase of true dysphagia—it is only a diminution of the painful sensation. It is not clear exactly how the pain-sensing fibers are excited. You can distinguish two kinds of esophageal pain: mucosal and muscular. Mucosal pain always signifies inflammation of the mucosa. Mucosal pain may be related to the composition of the bolus so it is not the motion of the esophagus that excites the pain. With muscular pain, the pain sensation may be due to distension or stretch of the muscular walls or to transient ischemia of the muscle.

The Specific Features of Odynophagia

The Character of Odynophagia

You can usually distinguish between pain of mucosal origin and pain of muscular origin from the character of the pain. Mucosal pain is usually described as sharp or burning. A patient once described it to me as "bright." I have found that a useful term to offer to patients. Muscular pain is usually described as "cramping" or "squeezing," and it seems to have a duller or less describable character, though it is not necessarily less intense. The pain of odynophagia is often limited to the period immediately after a swallow; it may persist to a minor degree in the absence of swallowing as well but it is always intensified just after swallowing.

The Location of Odynophagia

The pain in odynophagia is located in the same place as the sensation of dysphagia (Fig. 2-4). When the cramping or squeezing pain of muscular origin persists between swallows it may be confused with the pain of cardiac ischemia because of the similarity in the locations of pains of cardiac and esophageal origin. These locations are so similar that the distinction can be difficult. Pain in both states may be perceived in the anterior chest and in the anterior neck or in the back, and esophageal pain can even radiate to the shoulders. I have never seen esophageal pain project to the forearms or hands, and so such a projection of a pain of characteristic quality strongly suggests to me that the pain is of some other origin. When a pain with the bright or sharp character of mucosal pain is sharply localized, so that the patient can put one finger on the locus, an esophageal ulcer is usually the cause.

The Chronology of Odynophagia

Odynophagia of both mucosal and muscular origins usually has a very clear *onset* that a patient can identify accurately because this is an abnormal sensation. Because the causes of odynophagia are usually fairly stable, the pain, once developed, does not show notable exacerbations and remissions. It is present with every swallow. With pain of mucosal origin the degree of pain reflects the degree of inflammation. As the lesion advances or regresses the pain advances or regresses. Odynophagia of muscular origin usually represents a fairly constant abnormality, so that the symptom, once established, does not exhibit spontaneous exacerbations and remissions, although it is characteristically variable from day to day, from meal to meal, and from swallow to swallow.

Aggravating Factors in Odynophagia

Painful swallowing due to mucosal inflammation is frequently made worse by swallowing certain things, so you should ask about them specifically. The worst offenders are certain fruit juices (especially reconstituted frozen orange juice) and foods seasoned with hot peppers. The effect of fruit juices is due in part to the acidity of the juice but probably also to other unidentified substances in fruit juices. In food containing hot peppers, capsaicin (the substance that causes the "hotness") is probably responsible. It gains direct access through the damaged epithelium to pain fibers that it excites directly. Coffee is also a common offender and any hot beverage can cause pain when mucosal inflammation is severe. When the inflammation is particularly severe almost anything swallowed induces pain.

Patients with the cramping pain of muscular origin associated with esophageal spasm sometimes note aggravation of the pain when they drink very cold beverages and the pain may seem worse with swallowing poorly chewed solids, as would be expected since the pain arises from muscle contractions.

Relieving Factors in Odynophagia

Patients with pain of mucosal origin commonly take antacids or drink milk to seek relief. These measures are usually only moderately effective, if at all, because odynophagia usually represents extensive or deep-seated inflammation. Such patients avoid the aggravating beverages and foods. With pain of muscular origin patients try many things and do not find clear relief with any.

Associated Symptoms in Odynophagia

Weight loss is nearly always present in odynophagia of mucosal origin because the pain, which is impossible to avoid, is usually so severe that it inhibits eating. Pain of muscular origin is not so regularly associated with weight loss, unless it is unusually severe. Nausea and vomiting are rare in association with both forms of odynophagia.

HEARTBURN

The Origins of Heartburn

The sensation called *heartburn* differs from odynophagia in its character and its chronology. Patients with heartburn may also have odynophagia but the two symptoms are clearly different and they call to mind processes that are different. The sensation called heartburn represents chronic mucosal inflammation due to gastroesophageal reflux, which itself is chronic. Heartburn can be confused with other kinds of pain, especially angina pectoris, so you need to explore its specific features carefully.

The Specific Features of Heartburn

The Character of Heartburn

Heartburn is the word that is nearly always used in the United States to name the symptom and almost everyone thinks he understands what sensation the term represents without further description. Still, occasional patients with heartburn do not use that word but only complain of a pain or an unusual feeling. Whether or not the patient calls it heartburn, you should get him to describe it so you know what he is talking about. Such a description is sometimes hard to get. Although many such patients describe the feeling as burning in character, some describe it as a sour or gassy feeling, or call it a "sour stomach" or "indigestion." I presume that this is the feeling called *dyspepsia* or *pyrosis* in countries where those terms are used. Often no words seem really adequate to describe the sensation. It is helpful, though, for patients to reject terms that you offer like *sharp, knifelike, cramping,* and *squeezing,* even though they may accept *burning* and *sour* as not wholly adequate. The pain seems to be quite different in character from odynophagia, the bright pain of acute mucosal inflammation, but I do not know why.

The severity of heartburn does not reflect the extent or intensity of the chronic inflammation. It is a common observation that patients with a minimal esophagitis complain bitterly, while others with very mild heartburn may have very extensive or severe chronic inflammation. This lack of correlation between the severity of the symptom and that of the disease may indicate either that there is great variability in the sensory innervation of the distal esophageal mucosa or that patients differ in their awareness of pain in general; it may be that those who readily perceive the pain successfully find ways to treat the esophagitis, like taking antacids, while those who are less bothered do less about it and so develop more extensive disease.

Location of Heartburn

The location of the sensation is rather more consistent than is that of the other kinds of esophageal pain (Fig. 2-4). This may be because the inflammation in reflux esophagitis usually involves no more than the distal one-half of the esophagus. The sensation is always perceived anteriorly, usually over a rather large area centered over the xiphoid process, though it is sometimes focused in the midline of the epigastrium. I have rarely seen the pain from esophagitis centered very far toward the umbilicus or very far away from the midline. The sensation commonly radiates toward the suprasternal notch. It is only rarely felt in the back.

The Chronology of Heartburn

Occasional heartburn is a nearly universal experience so that patients will rarely be able to fix a specific time when it started. The symptom is chronic but inconstant. Exacerbations and remissions are nearly always present. Characteristically, patients volunteer that exacerbations and remissions correlate with practices that relate to aggravating and relieving factors.

Aggravating Factors in Heartburn

Because the symptom arises from gastroesophageal reflux, any factor that promotes such reflux aggravates the symptom. Recumbency does so because of the effect of gravity on fluid flow. Eating a large meal very commonly does so. This may not be simply a matter of volume, since large meals are usually fatty meals and fatty meals promote reflux; fats in the duodenum reduce the force of closure of the lower esophageal sphincter, probably through a reflex though the effect may be hormonal. In smokers a period of heavy smoking may aggravate heartburn; smoking has been shown to reduce the force of closure of the sphincter. Frequently heartburn is worse for a period after drinking fruit juices (especially reconstituted frozen orange juice) and coffee, and after eating foods seasoned with hot peppers; this effect probably represents the action of irritant substances in these foods on the exposed sensory nerves at the damaged epithelial surface. Drinking alcohol commonly makes heartburn worse. This probably represents an action of alcohol in reducing the force of closure of the lower esophageal sphincter. The taking of salicylates and similar drugs often exacerbates the symptom, probably because refluxed gastric content then contains these drugs and they further damage the already damaged mucosa. Vomiting usually aggravates heartburn, for obvious reasons.

Relieving Factors in Heartburn

Most patients seek relief by avoiding those exacerbating factors that they have recognized. Many also find that drinking milk or taking antacids helps. When a beneficial effect of antacids is denied you should ask if the antacids were in tablet or liquid form; antacid tablets are commonly rather ineffective, since the particles of the chewed tablet are not retained long in the esophagus but pass to the stomach before much dispersion or dissolution occurs. Some relief with the assumption of an erect posture is nearly always present. Belching seems to help many patients. Something about the sensation makes people want to belch, and they may swallow air in order to do so.

Associated Symptoms in Heartburn

When chronic esophagitis has been present for a long time or is very severe it leads to the formation of an inflammatory stricture. This produces dysphagia. The dysphagia may be so mild that the patient does not mention it, so you must ask about it. The occurrence of odynophagia usually signifies a focus of acute inflammation with the formation of a deep erosion or an esophageal ulcer. Weight loss is rare as a result of chronic esophagitis unless there is a very severe stricture that impairs eating. Usually patients tend to gain weight because they habitually drink milk or eat soda crackers to get relief from the heartburn. Occasionally the inflamed esophagus bleeds chronically enough to produce iron-deficiency anemia and the usual associated symptoms.

SOME DISORDERS CHARACTERIZED MAINLY BY OROPHARYNGEAL DYSPHAGIA

Oropharyngeal dysphagia may or may not be accompanied by aspiration of the bolus or nasopharyngeal reflux of liquids. These associated symptoms are the most valuable basis for a classification of oropharyngeal dysphagia; their presence distinguishes those causes that affect pharyngeal motility from those in which there is an obstruction to flow with normal propulsive forces.

Oropharyngeal Dysphagia with Aspiration or Nasopharyngeal Reflux

The presence of nasopharyngeal reflux and aspiration or choking with swallowing indicates that pharyngeal striated muscle function is deranged; such derangement may be due either to nerve or to muscle disease.

Signs of Neurologic Disease Accompany the Symptom

Because the programming of pharyngeal motor events occurs in the brainstem, disorders in this region can produce the symptom. The most common of these is *brainstem infarction* due to the occlusion of one of the posterior inferior cerebellar arteries, sometimes called the PICA syndrome (from the name of the artery) or the Wallenberg syndrome. The swallowing difficulty begins suddenly, along with signs of cerebellar dysfunction and, sometimes, Horner's syndrome. The dysphagia usually improves slowly, probably because of the subsidence of edema in the infarct, but it does not disappear entirely. A similar clinical course characterizes *infarction of the ninth cranial nerve* in diabetes, an uncommon event, except that the cerebellar dysfunction and Horner's syndrome are absent. In *poliomyelitis* involving the brainstem, a similar clinical syndrome can occur because of viral destruction of the motor nuclei. Here also the cerebellar dysfunction and Horner's syndrome are absent. Dysphagia is often a prominent symptom in advanced *Parkinson disease.*

Signs of Muscle Disease Accompany the Symptom

In *myasthenic syndromes* the dysfunction of the pharyngeal muscles may be the most conspicuous manifestation of the disease. The cause is usually evident from the involvement of other striated muscles. The striated muscles innervated by cranial nerves are usually affected the most severely. In the *muscular dystrophies* pharyngeal motor function is usually only moderately affected. This cause is also usually evident from other manifestations of the disease.

Oropharyngeal Dysphagia without Aspiration or Nasopharyngeal Reflux

This symptom quite reliably indicates a mechanical obstruction—compromise of the lumen—in the absence of abnormal pharyngeal motor function. Such an obstruction is more often located in the pharyngeal wall than it is extrapharyngeal.

Pharyngeal Lesions

Any mass lesion of the pharynx can cause dysphagia without aspiration or nasopharyngeal reflux. *Squamous cell carcinoma* and *tumors of lymphoid tissue* are the main malignancies of the pharynx.

Extrapharyngeal Lesions

Extrinsic tumors, if they greatly compress the pharynx, can cause the symptom. A *goiter* is the most common cause but goiters do not very often cause dysphagia. It is amazing how big a goiter can become without causing dysphagia. Dysphagia with a goiter usually represents substernal extension of the goiter with consequent esophageal compression. Any extrapharyngeal malignancy may cause dysphagia when it attaches to the pharyngeal surface or invades the pharyngeal wall. Such a tumor is likely to be readily palpable in the throat.

Cricopharyngeal Dysfunction

Sometimes esophagrams in patients with oropharyngeal dysphagia show a very prominent cricopharyngeus muscle called the *cricopharyngeal bar*. Some believe that this is associated with dysfunction of that muscle and that this dysfunction can cause the symptom. Objective evidence for this is scanty, but there are reports that cricopharyngeal myotomy relieves the dysphagia. It is also believed by some that such cricopharyngeal dysfunction can cause *Zenker's (hypopharyngeal) diverticulum.* This is a diverticulum arising from the posterior wall of the pharynx just above the cricopharyngeus. It is a common disorder, especially so in men past middle age. The idea that cricopharyngeal dysfunction could cause Zenker's diverticulum is logical in that a delayed relaxation of the muscle or a premature or very forceful contraction after swallowing could cause abnormally high pressures at this point and so produce the diverticulum by pulsion. The evidence for this is not wholly convincing, but surgeons now often cut the cricopharyngeus in the treatment of Zenker's diverticulum.

Esophageal Lesions

An obstructing lesion at the top of the esophagus can cause dysphagia that is interpreted as oropharyngeal. I have seen *squamous cell carcinoma* do that. The esophageal web associated with the *Plummer–Vinson (Paterson–Kelly) syndrome* also causes such dysphagia. This web is a thin membrane that partly occludes the esophageal lumen, usually located a short distance below the cricopharyngeus. It is strongly associated with chronic iron-deficiency anemia and it is more common in women than in men. It is not clear how it comes about. It can be difficult to demonstrate, being so thin that it is often hard to see in an esophagram unless a lateral film is taken, and it is often passed inadvertently at esophagoscopy.

SOME DISORDERS CHARACTERIZED MAINLY BY ESOPHAGEAL DYSPHAGIA

Antecedent or Concurrent Heartburn Occurs with the Dysphagia

Inflammatory Stricture

The fibrous stricture that forms in chronic reflux esophagitis is the commonest cause of dysphagia. The dysphagia is mild and intermittent at first and it progresses very slowly. The stricture is a reaction to chronic inflammation but there is no clear correlation between the severity of heartburn and the occurrence of a stricture. When esophageal peristalsis is normal, strictures may not become symptomatic until they are very narrow, but when peristalsis is disturbed (as in scleroderma or esophageal spasm) a stricture that is only moderately narrow can produce severe dysphagia. A clear distinction between the dysphagia of an inflammatory stricture and that of carcinoma is impossible on clinical grounds alone. For this reason all patients with dysphagia must have esophagoscopy and biopsy.

Schatzki's Ring

Schatzki's ring is a web arising from the mucosa at the squamocolumnar mucosal junction. It is always located within a few centimeters of the stomach. The exact cause is unknown but the ring may be a consequence of chronic reflux esophagitis, since the two are often associated. The dysphagia that these rings produce is characteristically intermittent and severe. Classically it takes the form of infrequent episodes in which meat or bread get stuck in the distal esophagus with perfectly normal swallowing between episodes. The episodes may show little progression in frequency; if they do they progress very slowly, over years. Large (or wide) Schatzki's rings are often found incidentally in patients without dysphagia. When they become narrowed to create a luminal diameter less than about 1.5 cm they are usually symptomatic.

Antecedent or Concurrent Heartburn is not Prominent

Primary Esophageal Malignancies

Both squamous carcinoma and adenocarcinoma of the esophagus often produce dysphagia without accompanying heartburn. This often occurs very early in their growth, probably because they interfere with the motion of the esophageal wall. The dysphagia progresses slowly and inexorably. Cure in both types of carcinoma is possible only with early diagnosis. For this reason dysphagia must always be investigated with endoscopy and biopsy of any suspicious lesion.

Extraesophageal Obstruction

Aortic arch anomalies, like arteria lusoria, a congenitally aberrant subclavian artery that compresses the esophagus against the thoracic spine, are rare causes of chronic dysphagia. Other developmental anomalies of the aortic arch may produce dysphagia.

Adherent mediastinal nodes involved in chronic inflammatory diseases like tuberculosis or sarcoidosis, or by neoplastic diseases like lymphomas, occasionally cause mild dysphagia. The symptom can reflect only adherence of the nodes to the esophageal wall to impair its motion, but more often it represents esophageal encirclement or compression. The dysphagia is usually mild, but chronic.

Mediastinal malignancies sometimes cause dysphagia. Esophageal dysphagia develops commonly in patients with thoracic malignancies like bronchogenic carcinoma, where the symptom can progress rapidly to complete esophageal obstruction. Any dysphagia at all in patients with such tumors signifies esophageal adherence, encirclement, or invasion of the wall by the tumor.

Motor Abnormalities

Esophageal spasm is a term that is commonly used to encompass a group of idiopathic disorders that are related but often distinguishably different. The basic abnormality is a disturbance in normal function in the smooth-muscled part of the esophagus. Five features may be present: (1) the progressive or peristaltic nature of the swallow-induced contraction may be lost so that the smooth-muscle part of the esophageal body contracts simultaneously in swallowing; (2) the force of the swallow-induced contraction may be increased above normal; (3) contractions induced by swallowing may be repetitive; (4) contractions may occur spontaneously, without a swallow to initiate them; (5) the force of resting contraction of the lower esophageal sphincter may be raised. It is rare to have all five abnormalities combined. Usually no more than three of these features are found together. The exact classification and terminology of these disorders is controversial. What is important is that all forms of esophageal spasm may produce dysphagia, though not always. Simultaneity of the contraction alone is commonly asymptomatic. The occurrence of dysphagia in patients with simultaneous contractions depends on the degree of obstruction to flow that the abnormal contractions produce. An increased force of the peristaltic contraction appears to be the abnormality most commonly related to dysphagia. The dysphagia of esophageal spasm is characteristically intermittent, varying from day to day, and it usually remains so without rapid progression. It may be made worse by drinking very hot or very cold beverages, by anxiety, by swallowing of poorly chewed boluses, or by eating in haste. It is rarely associated with much weight loss.

Achalasia or cardiospasm, an autonomic neuropathic disorder, is quite distinctly different from esophageal spasm, though esophageal spasm rarely appears to progress to achalasia. In achalasia there are two abnormalities: (1) the smooth-muscled part of the esophageal body does not contract at all in response to a swallow, or it contracts very weakly and nonperistaltically; (2) the relaxation of the lower esophageal sphincter in swallowing is either incomplete or absent. The combination of these leads to obstruction at the esophageal outlet so that the esophagus retains ingested foods and swallowed air and saliva. The obstruction is not complete, for patients often maintain a reasonable state of nutrition for a long time. Gravity causes some of the retained esophageal content to flow into the stomach. The volume retained in the esophagus is highly variable, from less than 100 ml to several liters, depending upon the degree of the obstruction provided by the nonrelaxing sphincter and the weakness of the residual contraction in the esophageal body.

The symptoms of achalasia are usually very characteristic. The dysphagia is mild, often described as a "full feeling" or a sense of pressure in the chest with eating. Regurgitation (quite distinct from nausea and vomiting) is common, especially at night. Patients may awaken at night to find food or fluid on the pillow. Regurgitated food or fluid is fresh or sweet rather than bitter from gastric juice. Weight loss is very slow and late in developing as a rule. These symptoms are insidious in onset and very slowly progressive. Some heartburn is often present, probably due to chronic esophagitis caused by fermentation of retained contents in the esophageal lumen.

SOME DISORDERS CHARACTERIZED MAINLY BY ODYNOPHAGIA

Disorders Causing the Bright or Sharp Pain that Suggests a Mucosal Origin

Esophageal Ulceration in Reflux Esophagitis

Severe reflux esophagitis often leads to ulceration. When odynophagia appears in a patient with antecedent heartburn you will usually find esophageal ulceration, but ulceration does not always produce odynophagia. When there is ulceration with an inflammatory or malignant stricture the patient is usually able to distinguish between the dysphagia caused by the obstruction and the odynophagia caused by the ulcer.

Infective Esophagitis

A variety of infective agents can cause esophagitis. Such infective esophagitis occurs often in the immunosuppressed state or in immunosuppressive therapy. The principal agents are the herpesviruses and *Candida*. The odynophagia is sudden in onset, very severe and unremitting, as would be expected from the cause. The pain is perceived very widely throughout the anterior chest (or back) because the whole esophagus is usually infected. Patients often have a "sore throat." Weight loss is notable, since such patients cannot eat much. Nausea and vomiting are not normally present. The pain is much worse with the expected irritant foods and beverages and less with milk products. Sometimes you can see the lesions in the mouth or pharynx as sores or ulcerations (in the viral causes) or as thrush (in candidiasis), but often not.

"Pill Esophagitis"

Many kinds of pills may lodge in the esophagus to dissolve there and cause a chemical esophagitis. The problem is common in the aged. The worst offenders are salicylates, nonsteroidal anti-inflammatory agents, tetracycline, and quinidine, but there are many others.

Disorders Causing the Dull or Crampy Pain That Suggests a Muscular Origin

Esophageal Spasm

A dull or crampy pain commonly occurs in esophageal spasm. The pain is an exaggeration of the dysphagia of this disorder. Classically, the symptom appears insidiously as dysphagia and progresses slowly to become painful. There may be long intervals without odynophagia but by the time most patients seek relief the odynophagia is quite stable. Although the pain is characteristically precipitated by swallowing it may occur independently of eating and drinking. In such a case you may easily confuse it with pain of cardiac origin because of the similarities in the character and location of the pains of these origins. The pain can be very disabling and many patients with esophageal spasm who have odynophagia lose weight because they have such difficulty eating. It is probably

Table 2-1. A Classification of Factors in the Cause of Esophagitis Due to Gastroesophageal Reflux

I. Factors that increase the frequency or volume of reflux
- A. Defective closure function of the lower esophageal sphincter
  - 1. Dietary factors
    - a. Ingestion of fats
    - b. Ingestion of alcohol
  - 2. Bad habits
    - a. Smoking tobacco
  - 3. Diseased sphincter muscle
    - a. Scleroderma
    - b. Other connective tissue disease
  - 4. Drugs that weaken the sphincter
    - a. Atropine
    - b. Other drugs with anticholinergic properties
- B. Raised or prolonged gastroesophageal pressure gradient
  - 1. Obesity
  - 2. Lying down after meals
  - 3. Taking large meals at bedtime
  - 4. Gastric outlet obstruction
  - 5. Delayed gastric emptying due to gastric muscle disease

II. Factors that increase the residence time of refluxed material
- A. Absence or weakness of secondary peristalsis (as in scleroderma)
- B. Loss of progressive nature of secondary peristalsis (as in esophageal spasm)

III. Factors that increase the corrosive nature of gastric content
- A. Hypersecretion of acid, in concentration or in volume
- B. Presence of bile salts in gastric content
- C. Presence of corrosive drugs in gastric content
  - 1. Salicylates like aspirin
  - 2. Nonsteroidal anti-inflammatory agents
  - 3. Some antibiotics (tetracycline, erythromycin)

IV. Defective intraesophageal buffering of refluxed gastric content
- A. Depressed salivary secretion
  - 1. In scleroderma
  - 2. In chronic usage of anticholinergic drugs
  - 3. In aging

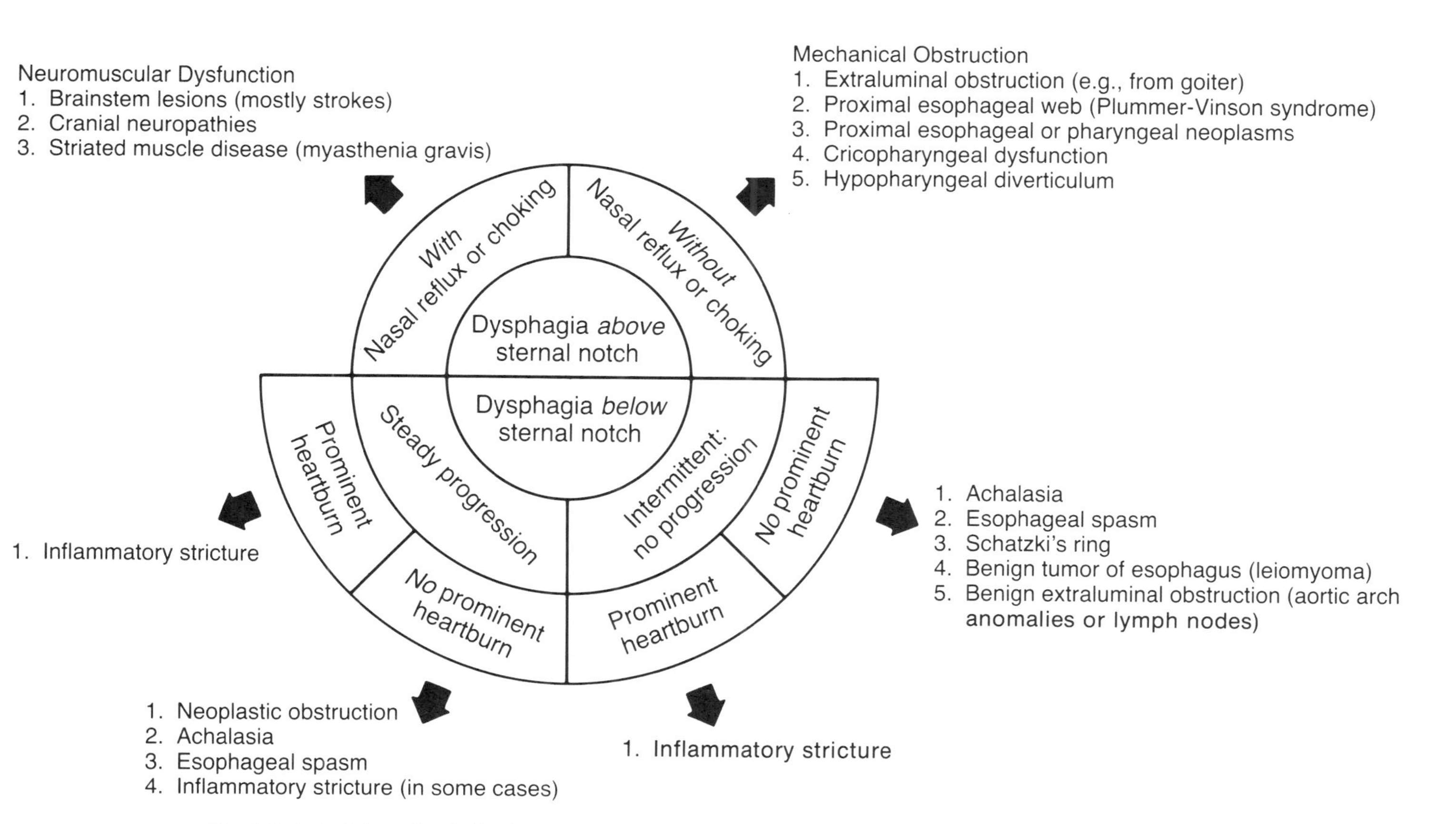

Fig. 2-6. A decision wheel classifying the causes of dysphagia on the basis of the location of the sensation (core) and other features of the complaint (periphery).

the increased force of the contractions that causes pain, perhaps from a consequent muscular ischemia.

THE CAUSE OF HEARTBURN

Reflux Esophagitis

The symptom of heartburn is quite specific for chronic esophagitis. The condition represents the consequence of the action of the gastric contents on the esophageal mucosa. Because some minimal reflux of gastric contents into the esophagus occurs in all people, reflux esophagitis can represent the consequence of several abnormalities: an increased frequency or volume of reflux, an increased residence time of refluxed material, an increased concentration of corrosive agents in the gastric content, or defective intraesophageal buffering. These mechanisms are presented in more detail in Table 2-1. They can frequently be identified in any single case and some can be corrected. In most cases several factors can be identified.

A DECISION WHEEL FOR DYSPHAGIA

Narrowing the list of causes in any case of dysphagia requires the consideration of relatively few essential clinical features, although the minor features discussed in this chapter are useful to support the process of constructing a differential diagnosis. The essential features are the location and chronology of the complaint and the presence of two associated symptoms, nasopharyngeal reflux or choking and heartburn. The use of these essential features is diagrammed in Figure 2-6.

3

PAIN IN THE ABDOMEN

INTRODUCTION

Pain in the abdomen is a very common symptom. Many different organs and processes can produce abdominal pain. If you explore all the details you will often be able to get quite an accurate idea of the source of such pain.

THE SPECIFIC FEATURES OF ABDOMINAL PAIN

The Character of Abdominal Pain

How to Get Patients to Describe Abdominal Pain

Pains in general are difficult to describe, but the description of abdominal pain is very important. The quality or character of abdominal pain can be very useful to you as you try to interpret such pain and you should explore the character as far as you can.

There are many ways to describe the quality of pain in the abdomen. Patients often use descriptive terms voluntarily but some patients will not volunteer descriptions. I find it useful to ask first, "What is the pain like?" The answer to this question may be quite specific like "a sharp pain," or the patient may refuse to answer, saying "just a pain." In either case you should press for a further description and it is always fruitful to do so. Do this by offering terms or descriptions from which the patient can choose. Ask, "Does the pain feel hot, burning, like a knife, like something sharp, like something moving around, like something squeezing, like something too big, or like a cramp?" Offered such choices, most patients will select one of these terms and you then can explore the description further. Sometimes after considering such a set of terms, a patient will refuse them all. Pains in the abdomen can be classified usefully in three categories: bright pains, dull pains, and undifferentiated pains. These three categories have different implications. In this chapter I use "dull" to mean "not sharp" rather than "mild": I use dull to refer to the *character* rather than to the severity of pain.

Bright Pains

The bright pains are those that patients describe with terms like "hot," "burning," "sharp," "knifelike," "stabbing," "sour," or "sore." Such terms denote a quality that most patients find relatively easy to describe and they will often select several of the terms that you offer as accurately descriptive. Bright pain in the upper abdomen is usually mucosal in origin. It signifies inflammatory disease although malignancy in a hollow organ can also produce bright pain, presumably because malignancy often has some associated inflammation. In organs that cause pain in the lower abdomen (the distal ileum and colon), mucosal inflammation does not produce a bright pain. It may be that the mucosa there lacks an innervation by pain fibers that can produce the sensation of that quality.

Dull Pains

The dull pains are those that patients describe as "dull," "squeezing," "cramping," "colicky," "like something too big," or "like something moving around." Such terms denote qualities of dull pain that patients find relatively more difficult to describe than those of bright pain, and they will usually select only one of these terms as accurate, and that with some reluctance. Dull pain is much less specific than bright pain as to cause. I think of it as arising from pain fibers that are not mucosal but deeper in hollow organs or in solid masses. Squeezing or crampy pain and pain that feels like something moving around usually represent an origin in the muscular walls of the gut. Such pain seems to represent some degree of obstruction to flow along the gut. Presumably it arises from abnormally forceful contractions above the obstruction. But such dull pain also occurs in nonobstructive disease like intestinal ischemia, for example. It seems to me that the fundamental cause of all such pain may be a relative ischemia of muscle.

When a patient describes a pain as feeling like something too big, he is usually right—you will usually find an enlarged organ.

Undifferentiated Pains (*Aching Pains*)

Pains that patients cannot describe or call an "ache" are undifferentiated pains. Of course some patients are not very verbal and they will not select a descriptive term for that reason. But when a patient of normal intelligence and understanding cannot find words to describe his pain adequately, it usually means that the pain is not arising from the mucosa or the muscle of the gut. This leaves the solid organs as the source. The pancreas, for example, is a common source of abdominal pain and pancreatic pain nearly always seems to be indescribable. Pain referred to the abdomen from the chest, as occurs in pneumonia or myocardial infarction, is also often indescribable, as is pain of abdominal wall origin.

The Severity of Pain

You should always try to discover the general severity of abdominal pain although the answers you get can be misleading. Very sensitive people perceive a pain as severe that other people might consider mild. Anxiety about the pain always makes it seem worse, while a patient who is preoccupied often perceives the pain as milder. An inquiry as to severity is a most useful way for you to open an exploration of the feelings of the patient about his pain. It can also suggest to you the magnitude of the causative lesion. You can get an idea of severity by asking what limitations the pain imposes on daily activities, whether it has led to lost workdays, for example.

The Location of Abdominal Pain

How to Get Patients to Locate Pain

The location of an abdominal pain strongly suggests its origin. For each organ the pain is usually most severe at its *primary site* and is variably perceived at *secondary sites* (also called areas of referred pain or projections of pain). A patient will usually volunteer to you only that location where the pain is most severe, the primary site. You must ask him directly about secondary sites. I ask "Do you feel the pain anywhere else or does it shoot or move to some other spot?"

Often the pain is perceived at secondary sites only when it is severe, being restricted to the primary site when it is mild. Also, in an exacerbation, the pain may appear first at the primary site and later at the secondary site. These generalizations are, however, not constant. Occasionally a pain may appear first or most severely at a secondary site.

The Meaning of Projection of Pain

The locations of sites of referral of pain are related to two factors. In many instances referred pain is related to a shared sensory innervation of various parts of the body. In other cases projection of a pain away from a primary site occurs because of the nature of the process itself. Thus, for example, when there is gastric obstruction from inflammatory disease at the gastric outlet the pain at the primary site (in the epigastrium) may be perceived as extending to the left upper quadrant.

The primary sites of pain in the viscera are usually immediately over or very near those viscera. The secondary sites due to a shared sensory innervation are quite specific and so they are very useful in interpreting specific sources of pain. These primary and secondary sites are shown in Figures 3-1 and 3-2.

Primary Pain in the Epigastrium

When the primary site is in the epigastrium the source usually is the pancreas, stomach, duodenum, or liver. Pancreatic pain commonly projects *straight through* to the midline over the lumbar spine. Pain from the stomach or duodenum infrequently projects through to this area, and when it does it usually signifies that the lesion is on the posterior wall of the organ. The sudden projection of an established epigastric pain straight through to the midline lumbar region always suggests that a chronic disease (usually a duodenal ulcer) has extended to involve the pancreas, for the midline lumbar region is the posterior

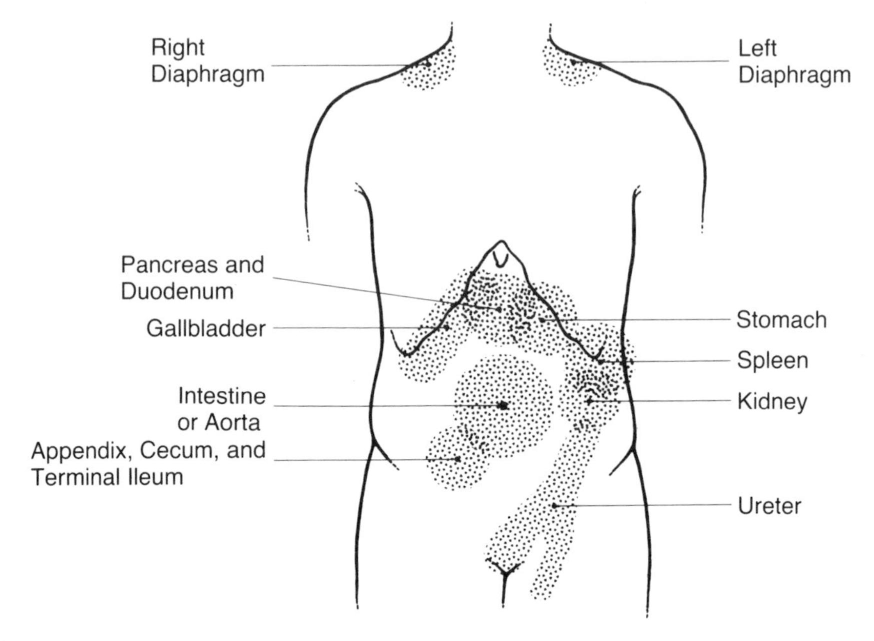

Fig. 3-1. Anterior view of the torso showing primary sites of pain from various organs in the abdomen. There is obvious overlap in some of these areas as shown.

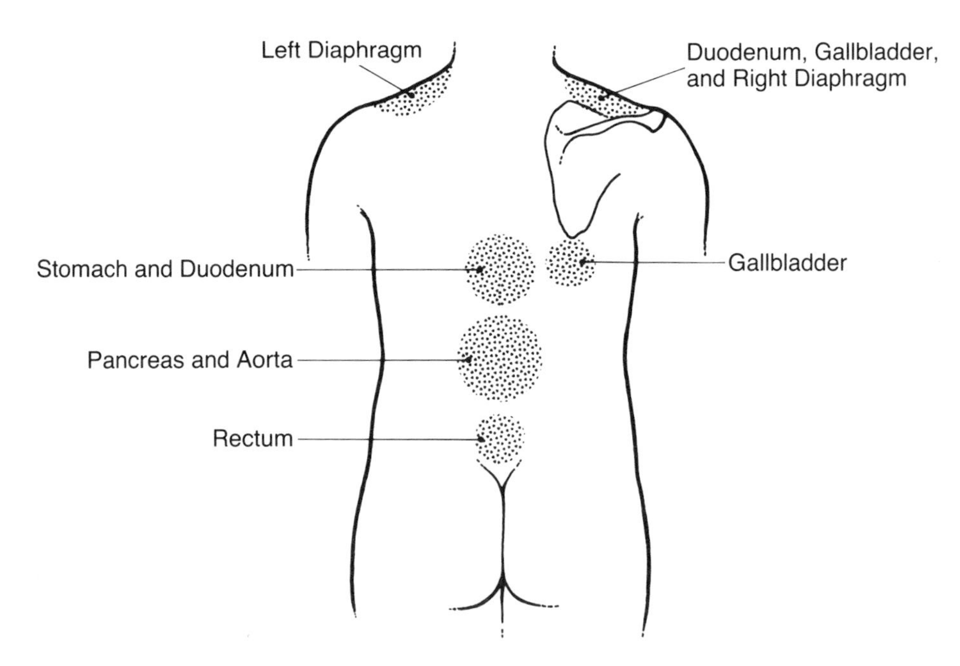

Fig. 3-2. Posterior view of the torso showing secondary sites of radiation or projection of pain from various organs in the abdomen.

secondary site for pancreatic pain, while the secondary sites for duodenal and gastric pains seem to be slightly higher in the midline of the back (Fig. 3-3). Pain from the liver sometimes projects into the chest, especially on the right side. This may occur when the cause is generalized throughout the liver (as in hepatitis) or when a localized lesion is at the dome of the right or left lobe. Pain of distal esophageal origin is sometimes perceived in the epigastrium. The pain of myocardial infarction sometimes radiates there and it may be felt primarily in the epigastrium.

Primary Pain in the Right Upper Quadrant

When the primary site is in the right upper quadrant the source usually is the gallbladder or duodenum, sometimes the liver, and rarely the colon. Pain arising from the gallbladder frequently projects straight through to the right posterior thorax in a discrete area just below the tip of the right scapula. It is usually said that gallbladder pain may also project to the lateral supraclavicular area on the right side. This is not common. Because this area is a common site of projection of pain arising from the right diaphragm such a pattern of referral always suggests to me that the diaphragm is involved in whatever process in the right upper quadrant is responsible. Pain referred to the right lateral supraclavicular area is often prominent with a right subdiaphragmatic abscess, for example.

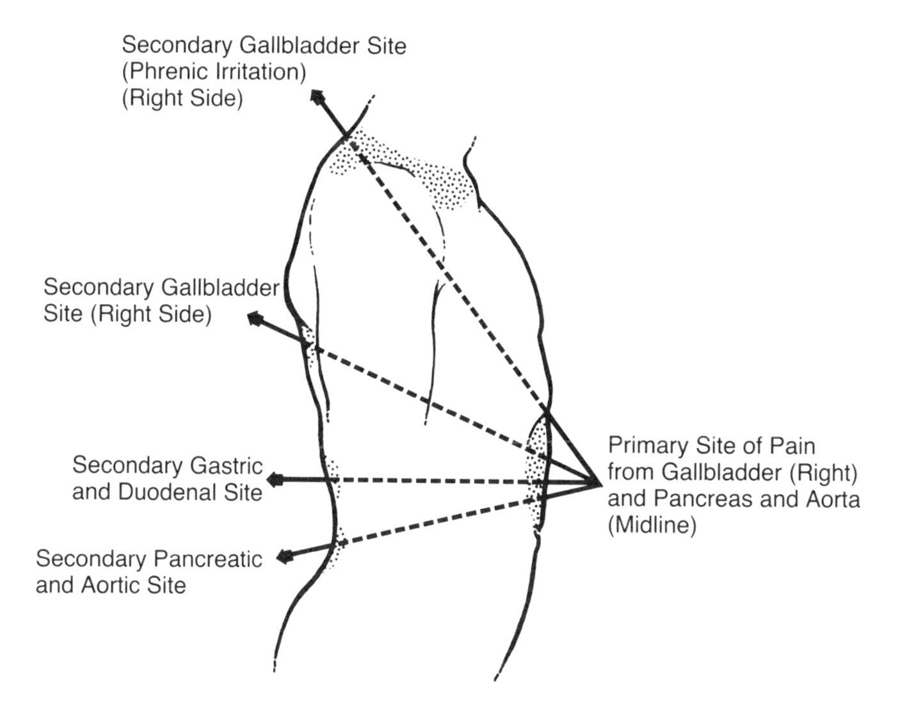

Fig. 3-3. Epigastric pains from the gallbladder, stomach, duodenum, pancreas, and aorta all project to the back by going straight through rather than radiating around the side. Pains from these organs do not always project to the back.

Hepatic pain commonly radiates across the upper abdomen and sometimes to the chest or into the right flank.

Primary Pain in the Left Upper Quadrant

A primary site in the left upper quadrant usually signifies a source in the spleen, sometimes in the stomach, and rarely in the left hepatic lobe or the colon. As in the case of the right upper quadrant, left upper quadrant pain is sometimes referred to the lateral supraclavicular area on the left and this signifies left diaphragmatic involvement in the pathologic process. This radiation is common in pain from the spleen, since that organ is in close contact with the diaphragm. Splenic pain also often radiates into the left flank. Gastric pain often radiates from the midline to the left. Left hepatic lobe pain (which is rare) can radiate across the upper abdomen and into the left flank, into the left chest, or to the left lateral supraclavicular area. Pain in this quadrant of left pulmonary or cardiac origin usually also occurs in the chest. Left upper quadrant lesions do not so commonly produce pain referred to the lateral supraclavicular area as do those on the right. This is because there is so much more potential space for expansion in the left hypochondriac fossa than there is in the right.

Primary Pain in the Periumbilical Region

When the primary site of pain is periumbilical you should consider the small intestine as the major source, less often the aorta and pancreas. Small-intestinal pain is diffuse anteriorly and frequently projects into the lower quadrants; it is not perceived in the back. Often pancreatic pain is primarily felt over a broad epigastric and periumbilical area anteriorly, and it frequently projects to the midline lumbar region posteriorly where it is often just as severe as it is anteriorly. Such pain goes straight through without lateral radiation. This pattern is very consistent and specific for retroperitoneal pain of pancreatic origin. Aortic pain (arising from an aneurysm) is usually felt over a more narrow area anteriorly and is nearly always felt posteriorly in the lumbar midline as well, commonly being more severe posteriorly. It is the general rule that significant projection of a periumbilical pain to the midline lumbar area suggests a source in retroperitoneal structures.

Primary Pain in the Flanks

Primary pain in the flanks usually comes from the kidneys, but it may arise as well from the gallbladder on the right or the colon on either side. Renal pain is often more severe posteriorly than anteriorly and it seems to extend from the front to the back of the flank by radiating around the side rather than straight through (Fig. 3-4). Sometimes musculoskeletal pain follows a similar pattern. When there is ureteral disease (as in the passage of a kidney stone) the pain radiates down over the abdomen toward or into the genitalia (Fig. 3-1). Gallbladder pain may be perceived quite laterally in the right flank. This location of pain may result from a lateral position of the gallbladder, this being one of the

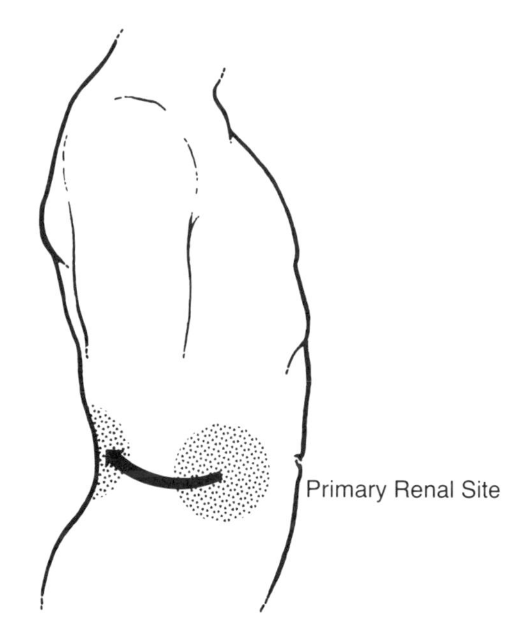

Fig. 3-4. The pattern of projection of renal pain with lateral radiation around the flank. The flared arrow is meant to show that the pain is often more severe posteriorly than it is anteriorly.

anatomic variations sometimes encountered. Pain arising from the ascending or descending colon may occur mainly in the flanks, but it usually spreads diffusely into the lower quadrants as well.

Primary Pain in the Lower Quadrants and Suprapubic Region

The colon is the usual gastrointestinal source of pain in these regions but pain of ureteral, renal, adnexal, and rarely gastric origins may be felt there as well. Colonic pain is commonly diffuse, radiating fairly widely in the abdomen; it does not radiate to the back unless the pathologic process has extended retroperitoneally, which is rare. Ureteral pain is usually easy to identify from its radiation obliquely from the flank to the genitalia. Adnexal pain is easily confused with colonic pain in its location, but patients usually feel it as being deeper in the pelvis.

The Chronology of Abdominal Pain

The Date of Onset of the Pain

When an abdominal pain has been present only for a short time, most patients will fully recall the date and details of onset. When an abdominal pain is more than a month or two old, the exact date and circumstances of its onset are easily forgotten. Precise dating of the onset of the pain is important in dating the onset of the process; also, asking about this is a useful way to get a patient to start talking about the circumstances of its beginning and its nature when it began. When a patient cannot remember the date of onset, you should offer him some recent landmark dates—seasonal changes, secular or religious holidays, political events or birthdays—to help him to remember. This may well lead him to tell you things he had forgotten—that it was first noticed or was particularly noticeable after a feast or after a fast, for example.

The Circumstances of the Onset of Pain

The circumstances surrounding the beginning of an abdominal pain sometimes suggest the cause. Patients will recall these circumstances voluntarily only if they themselves perceive the circumstances as being important. If your attempt to establish the date of onset does not yield a discussion of the circumstances of onset, you should ask if anything special occurred about that time. You should suggest some things that are appropriate—a forgotten injury or accident, a period of physical or emotional stress, an operation, the use of some drug of unusual nature or in unusual dosage, an unusually large meal or a period of fasting. Symptoms of inflammatory disease of the stomach and duodenum sometimes seem to start in periods of physical or emotional stress, or during periods of heavy dosage with aspirin or nonsteroidal anti-inflammatory drugs. Chronic relapsing pancreatitis can begin with abdominal trauma that may have occurred in an accident where the pancreatic injury was eclipsed by fractures, head injury, or coma. Bowel obstruction from adhesions or hepatitis from transfusion often follow long enough after an abdominal operation that the patient does not suspect an association.

Character and Location at Onset of Pain

When you are exploring the onset of a pain, it is important for you to find out about the character and location at onset, for these may have changed as the illness developed. The character and location of a pain do not change much unless the pathological process itself has changed. For example, a bright pain to the right of the midepigastrium (suggestive of duodenal ulcer) may have evolved to include or to be eclipsed by an undifferentiated diffuse epigastric pain in the periumbilical and posterior lumbar regions if the ulcer has penetrated into the pancreas. The severity of a pain also often changes as the illness develops.

The Progress of Abdominal Pain

Abdominal pain is not often truly constant; most abdominal pain is characterized by exacerbations and remissions. You need to find out whether the pain is indeed periodic, to discover the rhythm of its period and to discover patterns in severity during exacerbations.

You should ask, "Is the pain always there or does it come and go?" If the response is that it is always there, that does not mean that it is constant. Ask "Do you mean that you have it every day, all day and all night?" Almost always the answer will be negative. The commonest abdominal pain that approaches absolute constancy is that of pancreatic carcinoma. Constancy is also a feature of the pain of dissecting abdominal aneurysm and the referred pains of pneumonia and myocardial infarction.

When a patient acknowledges that his pain is periodic you must explore the periodicity. A pain that comes and goes with a daily or diurnal period is very likely to do that because its source is affected by a process that shows a diurnal rhythm—like eating, sleeping, and exercise. I call this a *daily pain.* It may not occur every day though, and I ask a patient how many days of the week he estimates that he has the pain. A constant pathologic process characterized by daily pain will usually manifest itself on at least 5 days a week. This is the case with many pains arising in diseases of the stomach, duodenum, and pancreas, less so in those coming from the colon and even less in those of splenic or hepatic origin. This is because secretory and motor processes of the proximal gut are those most likely to fluctuate with daily activities.

Other pains may be described by the patient as a single episode when, in fact, they are recurrent pains: He may have forgotten previous episodes if they occurred far apart, or he may be ashamed to tell you that he had the problem before and did nothing about it. You should always ask "Have you ever had a pain like this before?" This may reveal a pain that is characterized by discrete attacks and remissions. I call these *episodic pains.* With episodic pains you need to find out the frequency of attacks. Many causes of abdominal pain are episodic in nature, but the episodes may be weeks to months apart. Episodic pain suggests an episodic disease. The pains of relapsing pancreatitis and symptomatic gallstones, for example, occur classically as very similar attacks recurring at intervals of weeks, months, or even years. You must ask if the attacks are identical one to another or if they have changed appreciably with recurrences, and if their temporal spacing is changing. This will reveal to you whether or not the pathologic process is an evolving one.

With such episodic pain you should discover if *remissions* are truly asymptomatic periods or if they are periods when the pain is still present but so mild in comparison to attacks that the patient feels that he is well. In the periodic passage of gallstones, for example, the intervals of remission are usually completely pain-free. In gastric and duodenal ulcer, on the other hand, intervals of apparent remission are usually only periods of relative easing of pain, the mild pain in those intervals probably representing that of the more general inflammation which nearly always accompanies ulceration.

With episodic pain you should discover how the episodes begin and how they end. Ask "Do the attacks begin suddenly so that the pain quickly rises to its maximum, or does the pain take hours to develop?" Passage of a gallstone, for example, begins very suddenly and is quickly maximal, while an attack of relapsing pancreatitis or cholecystitis takes one to several hours to reach its greatest intensity.

You should ask about *fluctuations in intensity* of pain during episodes or attacks (Fig. 3-5). For most patients the term "crampy" implies such fluctuations but this is not always so. Some patients use the term to mean "squeezing" in character. You should ask "When the pain develops, is it perfectly constant or does it rise and fall in intensity?" The pain of cholecystitis is nearly always

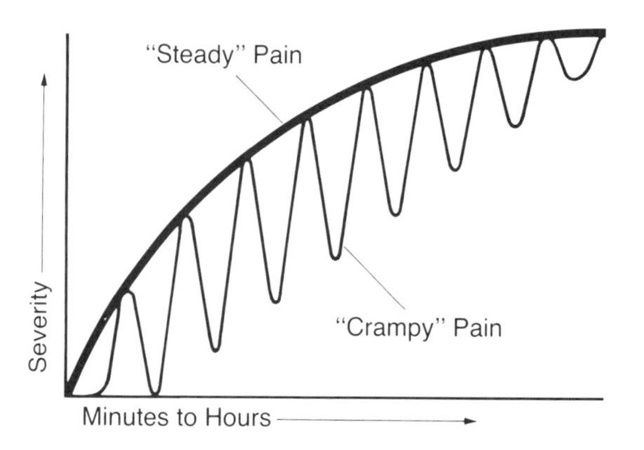

Fig. 3-5. A graph to show contrast of "steady" pain with "crampy" pain.

constant during attacks despite the widespread description of this pain as "colicky," as is also the pain of an attack of relapsing pancreatitis. The pain of passage of a gallstone, on the other hand, usually fluctuates during an attack.

Aggravating Factors in Abdominal Pain

Pains of abdominal origin are frequently made worse by certain activities and knowledge of a relationship can be very useful to you in interpreting such pain. The most important of the aggravating factors that you should ask about are eating and drinking in general, the taking of specific foods and beverages, the taking of medicines, defecation, body position, and physical activity.

When eating and drinking in general aggravate the pain, the pain is nearly always arising from the stomach, pancreas, biliary tract, small intestine, or colon. When the pain comes on immediately or intensifies within 45 minutes after the initiation of eating or drinking, the pain is usually of gastric origin. This may occur either because the stimulus to gastric secretion is very prompt or because some component of the food or beverage excites pain fibers in the inflamed gastric mucosa which it reaches immediately. When the pain does not intensify until an hour or more has passed the physiologic process is one that requires more time. In the case of pain arising in the pancreas or biliary tract this can be attributed to the fact that the release of enteric hormones in response to foods is slow. The effects of such hormones on the functions of the diseased gallbladder or pancreas produce the pain. In the case of the small intestine and colon the aggravation of pain by eating or drinking usually represents some degree of obstruction and it takes some time for the ingested foods to reach or affect the lower regions of the bowel. In intestinal ischemia the pain is always clearly precipitated by eating and it is usually very severe, but undifferentiated in character.

Often patients will have noticed that specific foods and beverages aggravate the pain. This is especially true in inflammatory disease of the stomach and duodenum. The most common offenders in such cases are coffee, alcohol, hot spicy foods, and fruit juices. You should ask about specific foods—Mexican or

Italian foods, pizza, and specific fruit juices. Reconstituted frozen orange juice is a very common offender. Prompt exacerbation of a bright pain in an appropriate location with the ingestion of such things is classical in gastritis and gastric ulcer, and it is present in some cases of duodenal ulcer. In some cases of pain due to partial distal small-bowel obstruction I have heard patients complain that the ingestion of large amounts of foods with a high fiber content clearly exacerbates the pain. Some such foods are obvious, bran cereals and celery, for example, but patients rarely gorge on these. I have also heard oranges, mushrooms, and water chestnuts mentioned by patients with partial intestinal obstruction; these are foods that people may sometimes consume in large quantities and which they do not recognize as high-fiber foods.

Specific medicines may aggravate the pain of inflammatory disease of the upper gut. The most common offenders are aspirin, nonsteroidal anti-inflammatory drugs, erythromycin, and elixirs of various sorts (all of which may contain alcohol). The mechanism is the same as that in the ingestion of irritating foods.

Defecation may occasionally aggravate a left lower quadrant abdominal pain. You should ask "Does moving your bowels affect the pain?" Because defecation involves contraction mainly of the distal parts of the colon such a relationship suggests obstructive disease in that part of the bowel. Do not let patients confuse normal defecation with straining at stool. Such straining commonly aggravates pain of origin in the abdominal wall, in which case the pain is often located in some other part of the abdomen than the left lower quadrant.

Certain body positions often aggravate abdominal pain. The dull pains that occur in a partially obstructed viscus seem often to be worse with the torso fully extended. In pain due to an enlarged solid organ or a completely obstructed bowel or gastric outlet, pressure on the abdomen is intolerable, lying on the stomach is avoided, and "doubling-up" makes the pain worse.

Certain pains often prompt avoidance of certain body activities. In pain due to pancreatitis, for example, any activity that jars the pancreas is avoided. These may include walking, climbing stairs, and riding in a car, especially over a rough road. Sometimes patients will describe restlessness with pain. Patients unsuccessfully seek a body position that gives relief. This restlessness is fairly common but it is not specific. The absence of restlessness is often a feature of pancreatic pain. When coughing, sneezing, or deep breathing aggravate an abdominal pain it usually signifies that the pain arises in part from the abdominal wall or diaphragm or from some organ that is moved by diaphragmatic motion, like the liver or spleen. Pain of gastric origin alone is not often aggravated by diaphragmatic motion because the stomach is deformed rather than displaced by diaphragmatic descent. Pain arising in the abdominal wall is usually aggravated by coughing and sneezing more than by deep breathing.

Relieving Factors in Abdominal Pain

While patients may tell you a great deal about the things that they have observed that make abdominal pain worse, they are rarely very forthcoming about relieving factors. You must therefore make an extra effort to find out about them, for knowledge about them can be helpful in interpreting pain. Of course patients seek relief by avoiding the aggravating factors that they recognize, so in reviewing aggravating factors you will already have discovered many things that produce relief. Certain other things that patients do are positive actions, like taking medicine. It is important to know what patients have tried to get relief without success.

In getting at this matter you should ask simply what the patient has tried to get relief. Because he may not remember without prompting, you should offer him a series of matters to consider. These are eating and drinking in general, the taking of specific foods and beverages, the taking of medicines, defecation, and body position.

Eating and drinking in general do not often relieve any abdominal pain except for that arising from gastritis or uncomplicated duodenal ulcer. The eating and drinking of specific foods is also important in relation to gastritis and duodenal ulcer, when things that patients perceive as soothing—like milk products—often produce a particularly notable degree of relief.

Many patients with abdominal pain try common medicines to get relief. For upper-abdominal pain they commonly try buffer antacids. When these are effective the pain probably arises from inflammatory disease of the stomach or duodenum. Such antacids are sometimes ineffective in such cases, either because the dose is insufficient or because patients often use tablet antacids which may not be adequately dispersed or dissolved in the stomach. Patients commonly try salicylates; these are rarely very effective in relieving any cause of abdominal pain and they often worsen the bright pain of gastric or duodenal inflammation.

Defecation sometimes relieves left lower quadrant abdominal pain and this suggests that the pain arises in the distal colon.

The body position that gives relief is quite useful in distinguishing pancreatic pain from pains of other origins. The patient with pancreatic pain or any other retroperitoneal source of pain prefers to lie quietly with his back slightly flexed, often on his side, sometimes on his back. This position may relieve pains of other origins as well but less consistently so. Patients with pancreatic pain sometimes like to press a pillow into the abdomen, sitting up and doubling over to do so, but such a position is not tolerable to the patient with cholecystitis or inflammatory disease of the upper gut. Some patients with abdominal pain find relief with the application of heat to the abdomen. I tend to interpret relief by external heat as suggestive of an origin in the abdominal wall, but this is no more than a suggestion.

Associated Symptoms in Abdominal Pain

A few associated complaints have quite specific meanings and so they are useful in the interpretation of abdominal pain. The most important ones are weight loss, nausea and vomiting, diarrhea, constipation, blood in the stools, jaundice, and bloating.

Weight Loss

Significant loss of weight occurs in many gastrointestinal disorders. When pain is the principal complaint, weight loss of much magnitude is associated with relatively few disorders. Weight loss can signify a reduction in caloric intake, an increase in caloric loss, or malignancy.

Any intra-abdominal disease in which the pain is exacerbated by eating leads to weight loss. Most patients attempt to get around the problem by eating frequent small meals, by avoiding offending foods and beverages, and by eating soothing foods like milk products which are calorically dense. These maneuvers work quite well when the source of pain is gastritis or gastric ulcer so that weight loss is relatively slow and small in those disorders. A patient with a duodenal ulcer often gains weight because such foods generally relieve the pain quite well. When the source of pain is the pancreas or biliary tree these maneuvers do not work, so that weight loss is more severe. The most extreme degree of weight loss associated with abdominal pain is that which occurs in carcinoma of the pancreas; this reflects the combined effects of a reduced caloric intake and of the malignancy. An equally extreme degree of weight loss occurs in intestinal ischemia because eating anything inevitably causes pain.

Nausea and Vomiting

The medullary nausea center is activated by both somatic and autonomic inputs so you must establish that the nausea is indeed related to the abdominal pain by asking about a temporal relationship.

Nausea accompanies many causes of abdominal pain. It occurs with both malignant and inflammatory disease of the intra-abdominal organs but it is more common with disease of the upper gastrointestinal tract than the lower. It is rare in esophageal disease, very common in gastric and small-intestinal disease, and uncommon in colonic disease. Nausea also accompanies diseases of the solid organs and peritoneum.

Nausea seems to be particularly associated with distension of the gut. Thus the development of nausea during the course of a well-established abdominal pain suggests that an initially nonobstructive lesion has extended to produce obstruction.

In the enlargement of the solid organs nausea accompanies rapid enlargement more than slow enlargement. Thus, it is common with hepatitis and pancreatitis, but uncommon in cirrhosis and pancreatic cancer.

Diarrhea

When diarrhea accompanies abdominal pain it signifies disordered function of the small intestine and colon. Partial or intermittent obstruction can produce episodes of loose stools. The most common lesions that do this are carcinoma of the right colon and regional enteritis. In both cases the diarrhea is rarely of much magnitude; it is often so eclipsed by the pain that patients may not mention it.

The pains of gastritis, gastric ulcer, and duodenal ulcer often cause patients to take large doses of antacids with a consequent diarrhea if those antacids contain magnesium compounds.

Constipation

Constipation accompanies abdominal pain in some situations. It may be a sign of ileus and it occurs in obstructing lesions of the distal colon like neoplasms. In diverticulitis there is often some constipation with the pain. In the irritable bowel syndrome the constipation is usually more complained about than the pain.

Blood in the Stool

The presence of gross or microscopic blood in the stool in association with abdominal pain means only that the lesion is mucosal. It can occur with all neoplastic and inflammatory lesions. The absence of observed blood from the stool does not speak against such disease. Some lesions bleed only intermittently and the tests for microscopic blood are not infallible.

Jaundice

Jaundice accompanying abdominal pain usually means that the source of pain is in the biliary tree or pancreas. There are some exceptions. An episode of hemolysis, as occurs in sickle cell disease, produces both acute abdominal pain, and jaundice. Also patients with Gilbert's syndrome may develop mild jaundice with fasting or fever along with pain from abdominal disease that is not related to the biliary tract or liver.

Bloating

When a patient with abdominal pain complains of bloating he is describing the sensation of abdominal distension. This usually represents obstruction of the gut at some point and it indicates that the lesion causing pain is also obstructive. It may also represent an ileus related to peritonitis or reflex ileus from pain referred to the abdomen from a thoracic disease like pulmonary infarction, pneumonia, or myocardial infarction.

A SUMMARY—WHAT YOU CAN LEARN FROM ANALYSIS OF THE SPECIFIC FEATURES OF ABDOMINAL PAIN

Character of Abdominal Pain

What it Can Tell You

This information can suggest to you if the origin is in the mucosa, in the muscle or at some other tissue level.

Reliability

Very reliable.

Problems

"Sharp" means "sharp" to some, "severe" to others; "dull" means "not sharp" to some, "mild" to others; cramping means "squeezing" to some, "rhythmic" to others; "stabbing" means "knifelike" to some, "momentary" to others. You have to make certain what patients mean by such terms.

Location of Pain

What it Can Tell You

This information can tell you which organ is the source of pain. The commonest causes of pain in certain specific areas of the abdomen are shown in Figures 3-6 to 3-11.

Reliability

Very reliable.

Problems

Primary organ-associated pain sites are not always quite consistent. The most common variants are: The *gallbladder primary site* is sometimes far to the right—almost in the flank; the *pancreatic primary site* is sometimes very high in

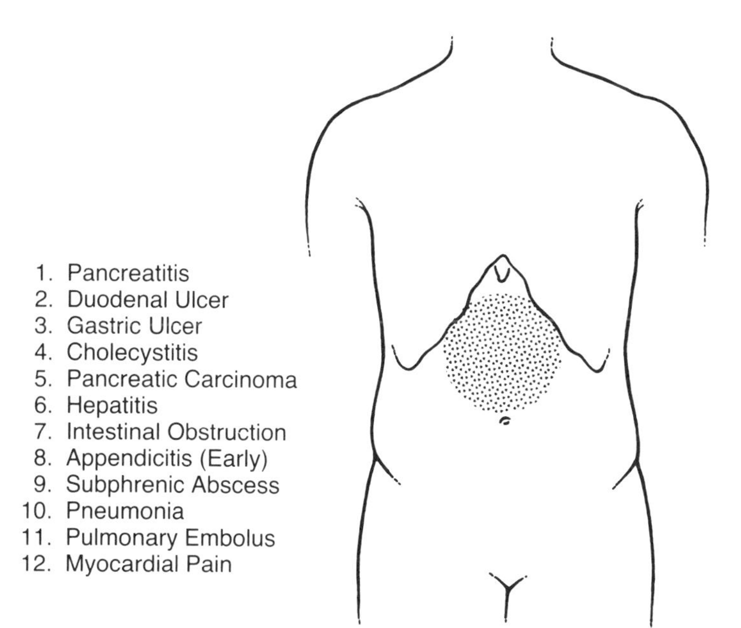

Fig. 3-6. The most common causes of pain in the epigastric area.

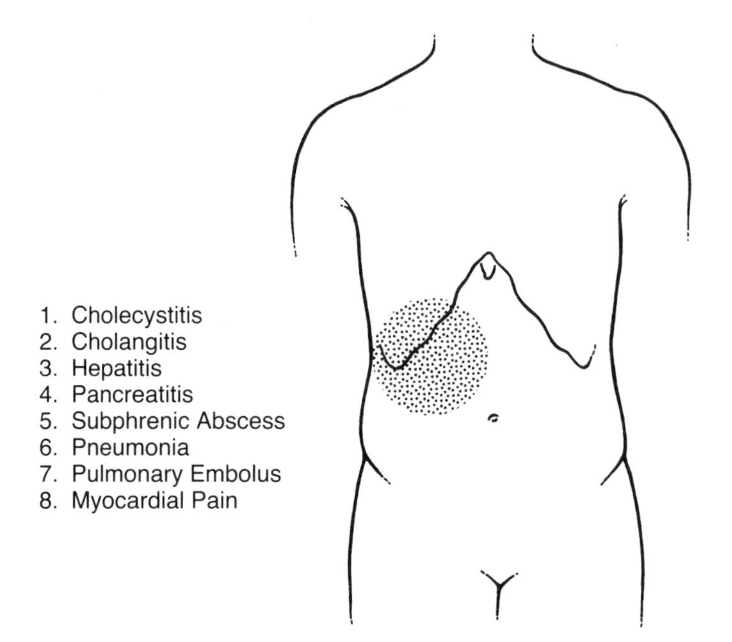

Fig. 3-7. The most common causes of pain in the right upper quadrant.

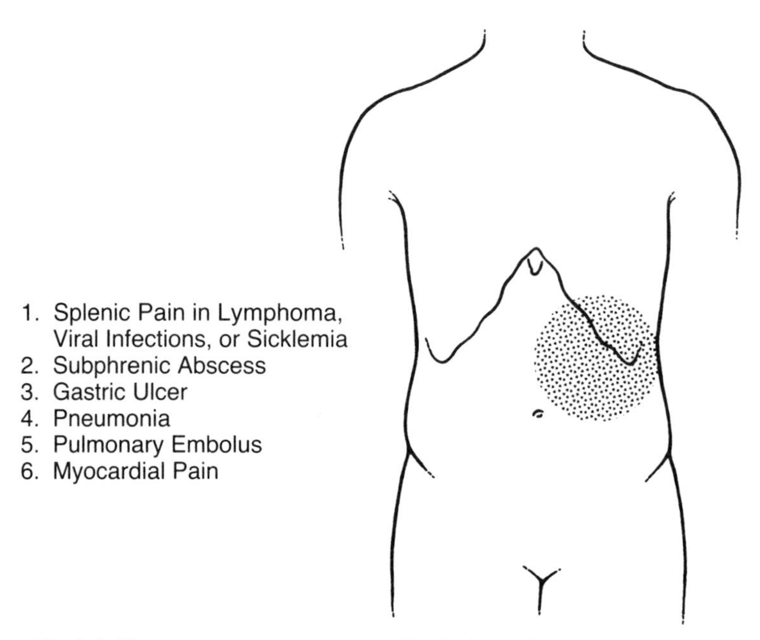

Fig. 3-8. The most common causes of pain in the left upper quadrant.

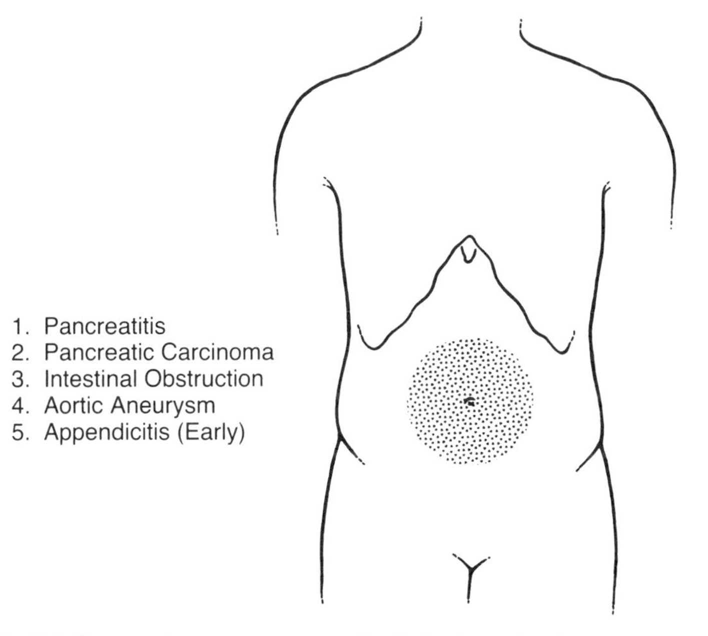

Fig. 3-9. The most common causes of pain in the periumbilical region.

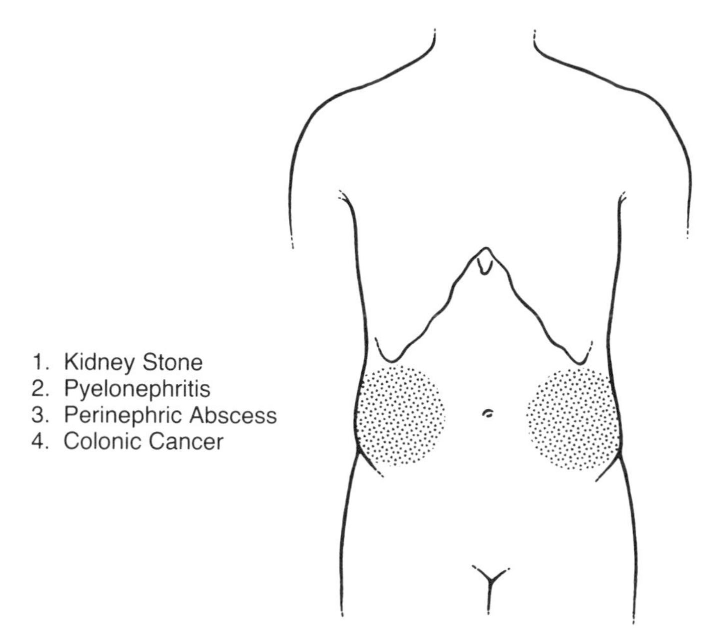

Fig. 3-10. The most common causes of pain in the flanks.

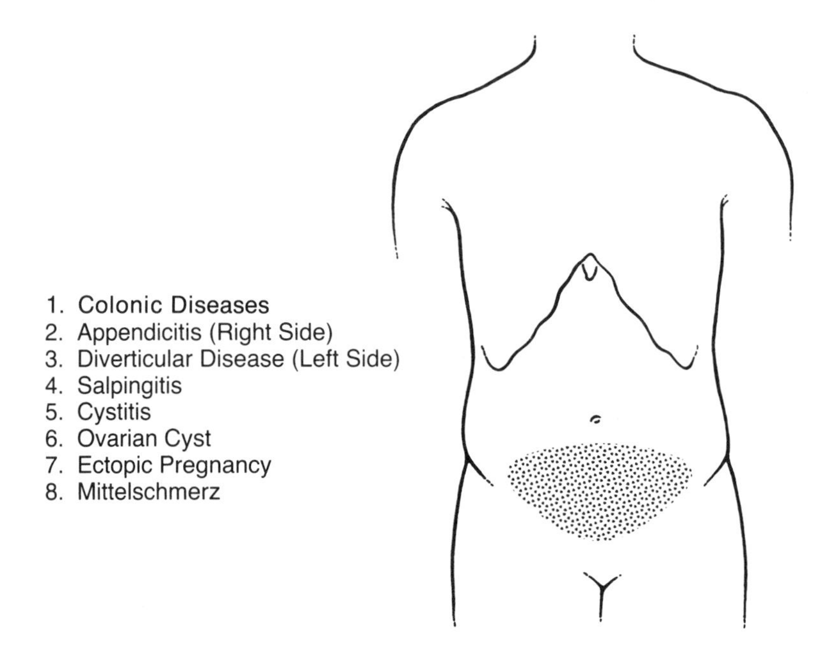

Fig. 3-11. The most common causes of pain in the lower abdomen.

the epigastrium rather than nearer the umbilicus, or even in the left upper quadrant; the *splenic primary site* is sometimes very far to the left, even posterior. *Secondary organ-related pain sites* are only sometimes involved. When they are it is very helpful; when they are not that fact does not exclude the organ that you suspect from the primary site. Certain locations are very suggestive of specific diseases.

Chronology of Abdominal Pain

What it Can Tell You

This information can tell you the nature of the progression of the pathologic process. The progress of the symptom accurately reflects the progress of the process.

Reliability

Very reliable.

Problems

Patients often cannot recall remote events well. You have to help them by offering secular or religious holidays or other special events when you want the remote chronology of the pain. Patients may not tell you of previous episodes of the pain unless you ask them.

Aggravating Factors in Abdominal Pain

What They Can Tell You

This information can support what you have already decided about the mucosal or muscular (or other) origin of the pain and the organ of origin.

Reliability

Very reliable.

Problems

Patients usually volunteer only the most notable aggravating factors and only then when the aggravation is severe. You have to ask about all the factors that you can think of to ask about. Positive answers are very helpful; negative answers are relatively useless. The pain of gastric ulcer, for example, is not always made worse by eating spicy foods.

Relieving Factors in Abdominal Pain

What They Can Tell You

This information can support what you have already concluded about the mucosal, muscular (or other) origin of the pain and the organ of origin.

Reliability

Very reliable.

Problems

Patients will rarely tell you how they get relief from the pain: You have to ask. Patients will almost never tell you what they have tried that did not work yet this can be very useful to you as you interpret the pain. Positive answers are very helpful; negative answers are less so.

Associated Symptoms in Abdominal Pain

What They Can Tell You

This information can support what you have already concluded about the organ of origin.

Reliability

Only moderately reliable.

Problems

Associated symptoms have inconsistent meanings. For example, some people get nauseated very easily, others not at all; some people stop eating (and so lose weight) very readily, others very reluctantly; some people with inflammatory or malignant disease of the colon have diarrhea or constipation while others do not, or do not notice or mention it. Some people with obstructing lesions (perhaps those who wear tight clothes) complain intensely about trivial bloating while others (perhaps those who wear loose clothes) scarcely notice extreme bloating.

SOME COMMENTS ABOUT THE FUNCTIONAL OR IRRITABLE BOWEL SYNDROME

Many patients with abdominal pain of undiscovered origin receive a diagnosis of the functional or irritable bowel syndrome. I have not considered this syndrome in this chapter until now, largely because the application of bedside logic cannot often point specifically to such a diagnosis. The reason is that the syndrome is only vaguely defined in terms of the symptoms and lacks any definition whatsoever in functional or structural terms. Indeed, the entity is undefined, and so it cannot be shown to exist and the diagnosis cannot be made logically. Still, many experienced clinicians use the term to describe a situation found in certain patients with abdominal pain and other gastrointestinal symptoms that cannot be explained in any other way, attributing the symptom-complex to emotional stress or anxiety.

The syndrome is characterized mainly by chronic abdominal pain. The *character* of the pain is nearly always described in terms that denote pain of dull character, like cramping, squeezing or colicky. The *location* of the pain is more in the lower quadrants, perhaps more on the left than the right, but it may be quite generalized. It does not radiate to the back or more remote points. The *chronology* of the pain is perhaps a little more consistent. It begins in the second or third decades of life and persists for years. It is a vaguely episodic pain, the episodes having no predictability or consistency as to onset, duration, or severity. The pattern of pain in an episode is inconsistent. There are no consistent *aggravating factors* or *relieving factors*. The *associated symptoms* usually (but not always) include some alteration in bowel habit (constipation, diarrhea, or alternating constipation and diarrhea) and this may be severe. Nausea and vomiting may or may not be present. Weight loss is not usually present. Bloating is a frequent complaint.

It is commonly taught that there are certain bedside clues to the diagnosis of anxiety-induced abdominal pain. These include inappropriate affective responses during the interview or examination as discussed in Chapter 1, the keeping of a complex symptom diary, and your discovery of secondary gain. All these clues are fallible. Deciding what is an appropriate affective response to the interview depends on many variables—your experience, the emotional volatility of the patient, and the character of the interview. Patients who are naturally compulsive or introspective may keep symptom diaries. And the discovery of secondary gain—the fact that some limitation of activity imposed by the pain is in fact the avoidance of an unconsciously undesired responsibility on the part of the patient—can require a very extensive probing and careful interpretation of patients' attitudes to themselves and to their diseases.

Those who make this diagnosis do so when they can find no other explanation for the symptoms. It is thus a diagnosis of exclusion. Of course what you look for depends upon what you think of to look for.

There is an intellectual trap in this. As soon as you have named a disease ("made a diagnosis") not only do you stop thinking of other possible explanations for symptoms but you also begin to think that you understand the process denoted by the diagnostic term you have chosen. Thus to make this diagnosis is to risk self-delusion, and worse, to risk missing another diagnosis that you didn't think of.

I do not deny that there are patients with chronic abdominal pain and altered bowel habit that defy analysis. I know perfectly well that emotional stress and anxiety can produce these symptoms, for that has been the nearly universal experience of every normal but terrified school child or soldier. I know also that the physiologic mechanism of this effect is not known. It seems to me that when anxiety seems to explain symptoms you should simply say so, calling them *anxiety-related symptoms.* To use a term like the *functional bowel syndrome* is to risk creating a defined disease where none exists.

I have seen many errors committed by physicians who made a diagnosis of the functional bowel syndrome too hastily. You may avoid such errors if you avoid thinking that abdominal pain has its origin in chronic anxiety when:

1. The pain is undifferentiated or indescribable as discussed above.
2. The pain is focused over a primary organ-related site of pain.
3. The pain radiates to the back or chest.
4. The pain began after the age of 25 years.
5. The pain is clearly made much worse by eating.
6. The pain is accompanied by more than occasional nausea and vomiting.
7. The pain is accompanied by any weight loss.
8. The pain is distinctly episodic with attacks and remissions lasting days or weeks.
9. The pain shows clear progression in severity or frequency of attacks.

4

DIARRHEA

INTRODUCTION

Diarrhea is a common symptom with many causes. Many diarrheal illnesses are acute, moderate, brief, and self-limited; these may not bring a patient to a physician. The physician deals mainly with more severe, prolonged or recurrent diarrhea. That is the main subject of this chapter.

Diarrhea has many causes and classifications of diarrhea are complex. A stereotyped approach to diagnosis, a routine series of laboratory and radiographic examinations, is not without merit but the use of these tests with a logic based on the specific features of the illness can make the diagnostic process much more efficient.

What Patients Mean When They Complain of Diarrhea

Diarrhea can mean different things to different people. The term can indicate increased frequency of defecation, increased volume of stool, increased fluidity of stool or abnormal sensations in defecation. These may all occur together but often they do not. Because these separate elements of the complaint of diarrhea signify slightly different things, you must always ask specifically about stool frequency, stool volume, stool consistency, and defecatory sensations to be able to explore the symptoms logically.

There is no problem in defining diarrhea when it is severe. The problem arises in defining minor degrees of diarrhea. This requires a definition of the normal variation in stool frequency, volume and consistency, and of normal defecatory sensations. A patient defines normality in terms of his own experience rather than some generalized layman's concept, since the subject of defecation is not a topic for regular social conversation. Physicians often suffer the same limited perspective, since it is not usual for them to discuss bowel habits in detail with patients who do not complain of disordered bowel function. Still, the matter has been investigated objectively to some degree so that the range of normality can be stated roughly.

What Is Diarrhea in Terms of Stool Frequency?

The frequency of defecation differs widely among normal people. Most people deliver a stool about once daily, some defecate twice a day and a few have three stools daily. I tend to accept the consistent delivery of more than three stools daily as abnormal. A change in stool frequency is more significant than the absolute frequency.

What is Diarrhea in Terms of Stool Volume?

The volume of the stool seems to vary with the diet. In populations that favor the usual Western diet the amount of stool produced daily weighs less than about 200 g. This value is widely held to be somewhat higher in countries where the diet consists of less highly refined foods than Westerners eat and Westerners who change to "natural" foods or become vegetarians usually note, or think they note, an increase in stool mass.

A definition of stool quantity in terms of weight is nearly useless to you when you are talking to patients, since patients do not weigh stools, but they can estimate volume. The volume of a stool of a given mass depends upon its specific gravity. The specific gravity of a stool must be variable, since normal stools may either float or sink. The water content of normal stool varies from 60 to 80 percent. The amount of gas in the stool also varies and this also affects the specific gravity. Accordingly the average daily stool volume (in populations on a Western diet) must be something more than 200 ml but probably less than 300 ml. In fact the average daily volume of the stool in normal people has not been carefully examined. I accept an estimated average daily volume greater than about 300 ml as abnormal. A change in apparent volume is more important than the absolute volume.

What is Diarrhea in Terms of Stool Fluidity?

The normal stool clearly varies enormously in its physical character, from a solid mass that seems to be quite resistant to deformation to a soft and plastic mass. People do not palpate stools but they look at them and so they will notice the *form* of the fecal mass. A normal stool is always solid enough to retain the cylindrical shape imposed upon it by the rectum and anal canal. A stool which does not do so can be considered to be abnormal.

What is Diarrhea in Terms of Sensations?

The sensation that constitutes the normal urge to defecate is virtually impossible to describe. It is like the sensation of hunger in this respect: We all know what it feels like but we cannot tell someone else about it. It seems never to be painful in normal people, but it seems always to be at least a little uncomfortable. Like hunger, it can be tolerated for a long time and it usually goes away for a time if it is neglected. Even in minimal diarrheal states, at least some of these features of the sensation are distorted. The sensation may be *intensified* so that it is sometimes painful; the sensation may be *intolerable* for very long, and it may *recur quickly* if it is neglected. These abnormal sensations are common accompaniments of many diseases that cause chronic diarrhea.

THE PHYSIOLOGY OF STOOL PRODUCTION

The delivery of a stool is the endpoint of a series of complex physiologic processes, many of which remain incompletely understood. A detailed discussion of the physiology of stool production would occupy a whole book and such a presentation is beyond the scope of this volume. It is necessary, however, for you to have in mind the general scheme of the physiology if you are to be able to interpret the symptoms of chronic diarrhea in a useful way. This section is meant only to provide the physiologic basis for a discussion of the interpretation of the symptom.

In the application of bedside logic to the complaint of diarrhea, I find it useful to think of the stool as the consequence of the actions of the series of organs and processes involved. This series is most easily and usefully considered in the order in which these organs and processes act in the conversion of what is eaten to what is defecated.

The Effect of the Diet on Stool Production

Most people assume that the character of the stool is affected by what they eat and that the amount of fiber is the principal variable. This is probably true, but the effect is not great and it is probably not fiber alone that is responsible, since high-fiber foods may contain other substances than fiber that can affect the quantity and quality of the stool. It is not quite clear that a tolerable load of ingested fiber can increase the daily quantity of stool very much. A major problem in this matter is the definition of fiber. Nutritionists define fiber in food as the residue that remains undissolved after a food is subjected to defined conditions of acid and alkaline hydrolysis—hardly a satisfactory model of gastrointestinal digestion. Vegetable foods contain a great many complex polymers that can be considered to be fiber and the fate of such material in the gut is unknown. Their effect on the character of the stool is a function of the degree to which they are reduced to simpler molecules, some of which might be absorbed but others not. These simpler molecules can affect the character of the stool through osmotic effects or as laxatives that act in other ways. The remarkable thing is that the gastrointestinal tract can handle the enormous variety of substances consumed as foods in a large range of volumes and still produce a stool that is reasonably homogenous in volume and consistency.

The Effect of the Secretory Organs of the Gut on Stool Production

The major secretory organs of the gut (the salivary glands, stomach, pancreas, and liver) produce a volume of about 7 L per day and the small intestine secretes about 3 L per day; variations in these volumes alone do not affect the quantity of stool because the secretions are mostly water which is removed from the lumen through osmotic equilibration across the intestinal and colonic epithelia. Deficits in the enzymatic activities of the pancreatic secretion increase stool volume because of the consequent defective enzymatic hydrolysis of the complex molecules eaten. This effect is not a linear process. These enzymes are produced in greater quantity than is required so that the character of the stool is not affected much in pancreatic insufficiency until pancreatic exocrine function is severely compromised.

The Effect of the Intestine on Stool Production

The intestine normally receives about 12 L of fluid per day, 2 L from the diet, 7 L from the secretory organs, and 3 L from its own secretion; it normally delivers about 1.5 L per day to the colon. This enormous volume reduction, 75 to 85 percent, comes about through both of the two functions of the intestine: motility and absorption. Motions of the intestinal walls mix the food the intestine receives with pancreatic enzymes so that the hydrolysis of susceptible complex molecules is complete. The intestinal epithelium acts as a semipermeable membrane containing mechanisms capable of the active unidirectional transport of specific molecules that are either eaten as such or are produced by digestion, such as glucose and amino acids. Water, the main contributor to stool volume, is handled passively by the small-intestinal epithelium; it follows osmotic gradients. The intestinal epithelium is a "leaky" membrane; it does not move sodium against a concentration gradient. Thus, the fluid volume delivered to the colon depends on the degree to which osmotically active molecules are produced by digestion and removed through absorption. If the removal of osmolytes is depressed the volume delivered to the colon is increased.

Defective removal of luminal osmolytes can have three general causes. First, the diet may contain osmolytes that do not effectively cross the intestinal epithelium. Second, intraluminal digestion may be incomplete so that large molecules, relatively inactive osmotically, are reduced to smaller molecules, more active osmotically but still not removable from the intestinal lumen through epithelial transport. And third, the mucosa itself may be diseased so that epithelial transport itself is defective.

The Effect of the Colon on Stool Production

The colon receives an average of 1500 ml of fluid daily and evacuates about 150 ml of water. Its ability to concentrate the luminal fluid is enormous because the epithelium is a "tight" membrane. The colonic mucosa moves sodium against a concentration gradient. The colon is not normally functioning at its maximal capacity, for the ileal input can be increased up to 4 to 5 times before stool volume increases. This concentration of the fecal mass is mostly the result of the active transport of sodium against a concentration gradient across the colonic mucosa and the passive movement of water.

In the small intestine the enzymatic conversion of solids to nutrient molecules that are absorbed in the small intestine (either by active transport or diffusion) is nearly complete by the time luminal content reaches the colon. As a result the colon normally receives very little nutrient material that can be absorbed except for sodium and water. A little material that reaches the colon is metabolized by bacteria to produce mainly volatile fatty acids, which are absorbed by diffusion, and gas, mainly methane and hydrogen, which are partly absorbed by diffusion and partly expelled as such or suspended in the stool mass. Thus the colon is the chief organ that regulates stool volume and fluidity.

The frequency of defecation is a function of colonic motility, mainly the motility of the rectum but indirectly the motility of more proximal colonic segments. The urge to defecate is initiated by receptive nerve structures, mechanoreceptors, located somewhere in the rectal or sigmoid colonic wall. The excitation of these mechanoreceptors initiates reflexes, mediated through the spinal cord but also affecting cerebral centers, that excite the variety of motor responses operating in defecation. These include relaxation of the internal anal sphincter (which is tonically contracted at rest), somatic movements associated with defecation, and contraction of the wall of the distal colon. The frequency with which these reflexes are excited depends in part on the frequency with which the rectum is filled, and so the frequency of the urge to defecate depends in part on the motility of the more proximal parts of the colon.

The urge to defecate can be resisted by conscious efforts, which mainly involve the voluntary contraction of the external anal sphincter, and conscious suppression of the somatic movements that are evoked by the urge. This capacity for voluntary resistance to defecation is also a major determinant of stool frequency.

A GENERAL VIEW OF THE PATHOGENESIS OF DIARRHEA

From the brief review of the preceding section you can readily understand that there are several ways in which increased stool frequency, volume, and fluidity could arise. Many diarrheal processes involve the defective mucosal transport of nutrients and water from the intestinal or colonic lumen to the blood, but this is never the sole process. The intestinal epithelium, when damaged or affected by many substances or organisms that can get into the lumen in pathologic states, is converted to a secreting surface, secreting electrolytes with water following osmotically. A similar reversal of transmucosal movement of electrolytes and water can occur in the colon. Since the volume, fluidity and frequency of the stool are all functions of its water content, any process that depresses water and electrolyte absorption or causes movement of electrolytes and water into the gut lumen alters the character of the stool in the direction of diarrhea.

Deficient digestion and deficient mucosal function get the most attention in the consideration of the pathogenesis of diarrhea, for these have been extensively examined in normal and diarrheal states. Abnormal motor function as a cause of diarrhea gets less attention, since motility, especially colonic motility, has had much less study both in normal function and in diarrheal states. Gut mucosal function and gut muscle function are not strictly separable in the consideration of the pathogenesis of diarrhea, however, for it is very likely that both colonic and small-intestinal motility are altered both by the volume and the chemical composition of the luminal contents. Also the reverse may be true, that the nature of motility affects mucosal function, since the mixing of luminal content may well be important in optimizing both digestion and absorption.

A CLINICAL CLASSIFICATION OF DIARRHEAL SYNDROMES INTO SIX GROUPS

There are several ways to classify the diarrheas. Most modern classifications are based on the basic physiologic processes that are deranged, like digestion, intestinal mucosal absorption and secretion, colonic mucosal absorption and secretion, and motor function. Because these physiologic disorders almost invariably occur together in various combinations in the patient who has diarrhea, I find such classifications to be less than satisfactory at bedside evaluation. Other classifications are based on the proximate causes: infectious diarrheas, pancreatic insufficiency, diarrhea due to substances that are ingested, or diarrhea of intrinsic mucosal disease of the intestine or colon. Such a strictly etiologic classification is also not wholly satisfactory at the bedside.

Still, it is necessary for me to refer to some general categories of diarrheal diseases for purposes of the following discussion. I find the following six general categories based on clinical presentations to be a useful scheme to think of at the bedside. You should not take these as sharply distinct or mutually exclusive clinical syndromes, but only as overlapping broad clinical classes or orders of the varieties of clinical presentations. Thinking through all of them can be very helpful in guiding you as you proceed in each case.

Ingestive Diarrhea

This includes the diarrheas due mainly to the ingestion of osmotically active nonabsorbed substances in foods and medicines. Examples are magnesium-containing antacids and sorbitol in low-calorie diet foods. It also includes the diarrhea due to the ingestion of lactose by individuals who are deficient in brush border lactase, and the ingestion of other disaccharides in those with the other much rarer disaccharidase deficiencies. The patients with ingestive diarrheas are not very ill and the stool is watery with a moderately high volume.

Toxic Diarrhea

This category includes the diarrheal syndromes due to the infection of the intestinal lumen and mucosa by agents that either damage the epithelial cells directly or do so indirectly through the elaboration of toxins which cause the epithelium to secrete electrolytes and water into the lumen. The infective organisms include pathogenic strains of *Escherichia coli, Salmonella, Shigella, Campylobacter,* and many viruses. This category also includes the ingestion of such toxins themselves, as occurs in some kinds of food poisoning. These diarrheas may be called toxic both because they are due in part to the actions of microbial toxins and because the victims are often quite "toxic." The patients are frequently very ill with nausea, abdominal pain, fever, chills, and weakness, even prostration. The stool has a moderately high volume and is watery. These are often self-limited diarrheas so that they are not really chronic, but they may last long enough to appear to be.

Maldigestive Diarrhea

This category constitutes mainly the diarrhea of pancreatic exocrine insufficiency. It appears to be principally the deficiency in pancreatic lipase that causes the trouble, since fat malabsorption is prominent. It also includes the diarrhea of intestinal bacterial overgrowth with colonic flora. The stool has a moderately high volume and is fatty in character.

Malabsorptive Diarrhea

This category includes a variety of entities in which the intestinal epithelial cells are chronically damaged in a variety of ways, like celiac sprue, tropical sprue, Whipple's disease, and giardiasis. The victims may be moderately ill with chronic diarrhea. The stool volume is moderate to high, and it is usually fatty in character.

Hormonal Diarrhea

This category includes a variety of rare entities due to the secretion of biologically active substances (hormones) from certain tumors. The substances act on epithelial cells to induce the secretion of electrolytes and water. The principal tumors that can do this are islet-cell tumors of the pancreas, carcinoid tumors, medullary carcinoma of the thyroid, parathyroid adenoma, and small-cell carcinoma of the lung. Thus this form of diarrhea is an example of a paraneoplastic syndrome. The patients are not often very ill from the diarrhea. The stool has a moderate to high volume and is watery.

Colonic Diarrhea

Many colonic diseases cause diarrheas which variably share several features: a moderately increased volume, the absence of steatorrhea, the presence of blood, and distorted defecatory sensations. The entities are heterogeneous. They include ulcerative colitis, ischemic colitis, carcinoma of the colon, diverticulitis, radiation colitis, the diarrhea of ileal resection (due to the action of nonabsorbed bile salts on the colonic mucosa to induce secretion), and anxiety-related diarrhea. This category also must include those toxic diarrheas due to organisms that particularly infect the colonic mucosa, like *Shigella, Salmonella, Campylobacter, Clostridium difficile,* and the pathogenic strains of *E. coli,* because these sometimes present the picture of colonic diarrhea with bloody stools.

SIX MECHANISMS OF DIARRHEA

Increased stool volume and fluidity represent an increased water content of the stool. There are six mechanisms by which this occurs.

Osmotic Equilibration

Water diffuses freely both ways across the gut epithelium following osmotic gradients. All gut epithelia except the squamous epithelium of the esophagus are very permeable to water. Osmotic equilibration increases stool water whenever osmotic pressure in the lumen is kept higher than that of plasma by the presence in the lumen of osmolytes that cannot cross the epithelium.

Maldigestion

Enzymes, mainly from the pancreas, hydrolyze carbohydrates, proteins, and fats to disaccharides, amino acids, and fatty acids to be transported from the gut lumen to the plasma by epithelial transport mechanisms. Disaccharidases located in the brush borders of epithelial cells reduce disaccharides to monosaccharides for absorption. Maldigestion increases stool water content when the complex molecules are only partially hydrolyzed to yield more osmotically active intermediates that cannot be transported out of the lumen by epithelial cells.

Epithelial Malfunction—Malabsorption

Epithelial cells transport monosaccharides, amino acids, fatty acids, electrolytes, minerals, and complex nutrients like vitamins by active transport, facilitated diffusion, and passive diffusion. Any mucosal inflammation or damage to the epithelium compromises these transport processes so that osmolytes cannot be fully removed from the lumen.

Epithelial Malfunction—Secretion

Epithelial cells also secrete electrolytes into the lumen but this secretion is normally reabsorbed so that net secretion is negligible when the epithelium is functioning in normal alimentation. Many substances, especially bacterial toxins, can selectively excite epithelial secretion so that electrolytes accumulate in the lumen in greater quantity than they can be reabsorbed. The osmotic effect of these electrolytes thus increase luminal volume and hence stool water content.

Exudation

The mucosa normally prevents macromolecules in the plasma, like albumin, from entering the lumen. When the mucosa is severely disrupted, notably by inflammation, albumin, and other plasma constituents, and even erythrocytes, exude into the lumen. There is usually not enough time or adequate mucosal function for digestion and absorption of these exuded elements so they raise luminal volume, and hence fecal water content, by their osmotic effect.

Motor Dysfunction

Contractions of the intestinal and colonic walls mix and carry forward the luminal contents. Both mixing and antegrade transport are necessary for normal digestion of macromolecules and absorption of osmolytes to occur. Theoretically, therefore, defective motility could compromise osmolyte transfer out of the gut lumen and so increase stool water content. Actually there is little evidence that deranged intestinal motility alone is ever responsible for diarrhea. Deranged colonic motility may be. The matter has not had enough study.

HOW THE SIX MECHANISMS OF DIARRHEA ARE COMBINED IN THE SIX CLINICAL CATEGORIES OF DIARRHEA

The brief review above of the pathogenic mechanisms that operate in diarrhea suggests that they rarely operate separately. For example, all diarrheas are, in part, osmotic diarrheas. Damage to the mucosa causes diarrhea through malabsorption, secretion, and exudation, depending on the nature and extent of the damage. The following consideration of the mechanisms that operate in the six categories of diarrheal syndromes may help you to understand their different clinical manifestations.

Ingestive Diarrhea

There are two kinds of ingestive diarrheas. Some result from the ingestion of osmolytes that are not absorbed, like sorbitol in some ''sugar-free'' foods. Hence these are purely osmotic diarrheas, and stool volume, frequency, and consistency vary with the quantity of osmolyte taken in. In other cases the intake of medicines or foods containing laxative substances that stimulate epithelial secretion is responsible for diarrhea. These laxative diarrheas involve both secretory and osmotic mechanisms. The stimulatory effect is dose-related so that the degree of diarrhea is also related to the degree of intake. In both kinds of ingestive diarrheas fat is absent from the stool because digestion and absorption are not effectively compromised.

Toxic Diarrhea

Many enteropathic organisms elaborate toxins that stimulate epithelial secretion. In some cases there is also epithelial invasion with consequent epithelial damage and mucosal inflammation. Thus the increased stool water content can represent several mechanisms: osmotic effects, epithelial malabsorption, epithelial secretion, and exudation. The mechanism of secretion usually dominates, however, so that these are mainly large-volume watery diarrheas. The effect on secretion can be very large so that in these nearly purely secretory diarrheas, electrolyte depletion occurs and dehydration is a threat. The ingestion of bacterial toxins in food poisoning produces the same kind of diarrhea by stimulation of epithelial secretion. In viral enteritis there is often evidence for epithelial damage and mucosal inflammation but the diarrhea is mainly the watery high-volume diarrhea that reflects epithelial secretion.

Maldigestive Diarrhea

In pancreatic exocrine insufficiency the deficit in enzymes results in incomplete degradation of complex food molecules to yield an increased osmotic activity exerted by solutes that cannot be absorbed, so that stool water content is increased osmotically. The maldigestion is most conspicuous for fats. The normal diet contains some hydroxy fatty acids and colonic bacteria can make hydroxy fatty acids from unabsorbed fatty acids that reach the colon. Hydroxy fatty acids stimulate electrolyte secretion by the colonic epithelium. Thus maldigestive diarrhea involves maldigestion, epithelial secretion and osmotic equilibration.

Malabsorptive Diarrhea

Any form of damage to the intestinal epithelium compromises the removal of osmolytes from the lumen and so increases luminal water content by osmotic equilibration. Brush border disaccharidase activity also suffers in epithelial damage so that disaccharides, being poorly absorbed, reach the colon where bacteria reduce them to volatile fatty acids and gas. This effect of disaccharidase deficiency is technically a maldigestion but it is a part of generalized mucosal disease, so that the mechanism of disaccharide maldigestion is one feature of malabsorption. Severe epithelial damage also causes exudation of plasma components. Thus malabsorptive diarrheas can involve not only epithelial malabsorption but also osmotic equilibration, maldigestion, epithelial secretion, and exudation. The volume of the stool, the degree to which it is predominantly watery or fatty and the degree of weight loss all depend upon the degree of epithelial damage.

Vagotomy sometimes results in a diarrhea that is malabsorptive in character with low-volume fatty stools. The mechanisms include a reduced effective pancreatic secretion because vagotomy changes the gastric emptying pattern and this destroys the normal correlation between pancreatic secretion and gastric emptying. Thus postvagotomy diarrhea involves maldigestion, motor dysfunction, and osmotic equilibration.

Hormonal Diarrhea

The unregulated secretion of peptide hormones, notably gastrin and vasoactive intestinal peptide, from adenomatous or malignant tumors leads to high circulating plasma concentrations of hormones that stimulate intestinal epithelial secretion of electrolytes and water. The diarrhea produced is almost purely due to epithelial secretion. The constancy of hormone production establishes a stool of consistently watery character, often in consistently high volume, and the secretory stimulation poses the threat of electrolyte depletion.

Colonic Diarrhea

Many mechanisms prevail in this heterogeneous group of diarrheas. In any form of colonic mucosal inflammation the damaged mucosa fails to absorb electrolytes (epithelial malabsorption), secretes electrolytes (epithelial secretion) and loses plasma constituents and erythrocytes (exudation). The severity of the diarrhea depends upon the severity and extent of the colonic mucosal damage.

In colonic carcinoma the mechanisms of diarrhea are not wholly clear. They may include changes in colonic motility that result from a partial obstruction (motor dysfunction) and the osmotic effects of bacterial degradation of plasma or blood constituents that escape from the tumors (exudation). Similar mechanisms probably explain the diarrhea of diverticulitis, which can also produce both obstruction and bleeding.

In ileal resection the diarrhea results from mechanisms that vary according to the length of ileum removed. When the ileal resection is short (generally less than 50 cm) bile salts, normally 90 percent absorbed in the terminal ileum, escape into the colon where they are deconjugated by colonic bacteria and then stimulate colonic epithelial secretion ("bile salt diarrhea"). When the ileal resection is longer the body bile salt pool is depleted so that bile salt concentration in the intestine is insufficient for complete solubilization of dietary fats. As a result, undigested fats escape to the colon. Thus the diarrhea of ileal resection can involve both maldigestion and epithelial secretion. The degree to which the stool is fatty depends on which mechanism predominates, a function of the length of the resection. Long ileal resections (more than about 100 cm) produce fatty stools; shorter ileal resection (50 cm or less) produce watery stools.

In anxiety-related diarrhea, which may include some cases of the ill-defined functional bowel syndromes, evidence supports altered contractions in the colon (motor dysfunction) which could well explain the low-volume watery diarrhea that is characteristic.

THE SPECIFIC FEATURES OF DIARRHEA

The Character of the Stool

You must explore the character of the stool completely. Patients are usually quite willing to describe the stool if you question them carefully. The features that you should cover are the appearance, the volume, and the odor.

The Appearance of the Stool

I begin by asking "what does the stool look like?" The answer is rarely very specific and usually is an expression only of its color and fluidity.

Knowing the *color* of a diarrheal stool is of some importance. Normal stools may be variable shades of yellow to brown, of course. In melena, the stool is *black* and usually abnormally fluid, but patients often fail to mention the fluidity, only the color. The *clay-colored* stools of obstructive jaundice are soft but usually formed. The very rare *silver* stool of ampullary carcinoma is also soft but usually formed. Diarrheal stools are often *green*, but that color has no special significance.

You must know if the diarrheal stool is *bloody*. This is such an important point that you should always ask specifically about blood—patients may not mention blood if they see it only occasionally. The point is important because gross red blood in the stool virtually always signifies a colonic diarrhea.

It is easy to get patients to talk about the *fluidity* of the stool and it is important to know about it. When the stool is very fluid it means only that the water content is very high, and this signifies many diseases that prevent colonic concentration of the stool. When the stool retains its form, that signifies a smaller increase in water content. Such soft or poorly formed stools usually signify a disease of lesser magnitude, but severe colonic disease that is limited to the left colon may also cause such stools. The stool mass normally achieves its cylindrical form in the mid-transverse colon, so that in diarrhea characterized by the delivery of stools that retain their form the function of the left colon is probably not severely deranged. Formless stools mean either that the left colon is being presented more than it can handle (the usual case) or that the capacity of the left colon itself to form the stool is compromised.

When the stool is formless do not be satisfied with only that information. The *consistency* of the formless stool can suggest much about the nature of the disease process. Because patients rarely volunteer satisfactory adjectives I offer suggestions. Stools that contain much fat are often describable as *floating, mushy, foamy, oily,* or *sticky,* and they are often difficult to flush from the toilet. You should specifically ask about all these features of stool consistency. If the stool seems to be fatty it points to maldigestive or malabsorptive diarrhea. Stools float because of the gas they contain, not because of the fat, but fatty stools usually contain gas.

The Volume of the Stool

The volume of the stool varies greatly among the different diarrheal diseases and the estimated volume provides a useful criterion in the construction of a differential diagnosis. A patient never measures his stool volume, of course, but he often is quite willing to estimate it. I ask "if you collected all your stools over a 24-hour period, would they fill a pint jar, a quart jar or more?" Patients usually overestimate volume, so if they say less than a pint I accept that as indicating diarrhea of reasonably normal volume; if they say more than a quart I take that as high-volume diarrhea. You can, of course, directly measure volumes but that is not readily done except in the hospital, and it must be done continuously over several days to avoid sampling error. It is a useful and cheap way to follow the course of high-volume diarrhea under treatment. High-volume diarrhea points to excessive intestinal secretion and it is especially characteristic of toxic diarrheas, malabsorptive diarrheas, and hormonal diarrheas.

The Odor of the Stool

Stools that contain much fat are usually very malodorous, but patients do not often volunteer to discuss that. Because this is a useful point in identifying steatorrhea, you must ask about odor. If you ask simply, "How does the stool smell?" you will usually get the answer, "Terrible." All stools smell bad to some degree. You must pursue the questioning: "How bad?" You should go even further: "Do you have to open the bathroom window or turn on the fan? Do you have to spray the bathroom after you move your bowels? Do you burn a candle in the bathroom after you move your bowels? Do other people at home complain of the odor?" By such a line of questions you can estimate the degree of unpleasantness of the stool and so you can decide if you must pursue steatorrhea as a possibility. If possible you should smell the stool yourself. Steatorrhea points to maldigestive and malabsorptive diarrhea.

The Chronology of Diarrhea

The chronology of the symptom mirrors the chronology of the pathophysiologic process. You should therefore explore the onset, the rate of progression, and the tendency to exacerbations and remissions.

Onset

An abrupt onset usually signifies a toxic diarrhea, or an ingestive diarrhea when there has been a sudden change in diet or medication. Ask "How did this begin?" If it was sudden the patient can usually date the onset quite accurately. When you hear that the diarrhea began gradually or that the start cannot be accurately dated, such an insidious onset should suggest to you any or all the other possibilities as to cause. Hence an insidious onset is not very helpful except to speak against ingestive and toxic diarrheas.

The circumstances of the onset can strongly direct you to the cause of the diarrhea. Patients often notice the circumstances, but sometimes they do not, so you must ask them about this. You must be specific. Ask the patient what he was doing when the diarrhea started; ask if he had any transient illness at the time, if he began to take or changed the dose of any medicine he was taking, if his diet changed then, or if he was traveling. When a persistent diarrhea begins during a trip, especially to a primitive area with a dubious water supply, you should suspect a toxic, malabsorptive, or colonic diarrhea due to an infective agent, such as *Giardia*. Of course, one can get *Giardia* at home too.

Progress

Diarrhea that is acute in onset usually progresses rapidly over 24 to 48 hours and this is characteristic of most toxic diarrheas. A slow steady progression (over weeks to months) is especially characteristic of diarrheas related to malignancies, either indirectly as in the hormonal diarrheas, or directly as in colonic carcinoma; slow progression also characterizes many other colonic diarrheas and many of the malabsorptive diarrheas. Diarrhea that reaches a steady state and has ceased to progress appreciably is characteristic of maldigestive diarrhea, but this feature also characterizes some malabsorptive diarrheas, some hormonal diarrheas and some colonic diarrheas.

Exacerbations and Remissions

Some fluctuation in intensity characterizes most chronic diarrheas. This is because the kinds and quantities of foods patients with diarrhea consume affect stool volume, whatever the nature of the pathologic process. The exceptions are those diarrheas that are mainly due to mucosal secretion, especially the hormonal diarrheas in which continued diarrhea in the face of fasting is taken as strong evidence for hormonal stimulation of secretion. When you ask if there are variations in severity you will not hear denial very often. You mainly want to know if the exacerbations and remissions are complete or minor in degree. If remissions are complete, that fact strongly suggests an ingestive diarrhea, for people usually do not eat the same thing every day and they may not take the same quantity of medicines every day.

Frequency and Diurnal Pattern

It is useful to ask about stool frequency and variations in diurnal frequency. Stool frequency generally parallels stool volume, and severe high-volume diarrhea can be characterized by nearly hourly stools. When the frequency of stooling seems to greatly exceed the stool volume in relative magnitude, suspect a colonic diarrhea involving especially the sigmoid colon and rectum. Both inflammatory and malignant disease of the rectum or sigmoid colon often cause the frequent delivery of small volumes of stool.

It is common to ask about the diurnal pattern of stooling when you want to distinguish anxiety-related (functional) diarrhea from other causes of diarrhea. It is widely believed that the failure of the urge to defecate to occur at night means that the diarrhea is anxiety-related or functional, presumably because patients do not worry when they are sleeping. This is not a fully reliable sign. I find that stooling is less at night in most diarrheal illnesses. The reverse is more useful information. If stooling is fairly constant night and day, the cause is probably not related to anxiety.

Aggravating Factors in Diarrhea

Many patients with all forms of diarrhea feel that anxiety worsens the problem. This is not useful information. The only important aggravating factor in chronic diarrhea is the eating of specific kinds of foods or the taking of specific medicines.

Relieving Factors in Diarrhea

Most patients try the elimination of certain foods, often illogically. You should ask specifically about this, asking both about what has succeeded and about what has failed. It is rare that a patient hits upon a successful maneuver or, when he does, recognizes why it works. Mainly the diarrheas that are ameliorated by changes in diet are the ingestive, malabsorptive, and maldigestive diarrheas. In ingestive diarrhea it is usually the reduction of lactose intake that is successful, but a patient may not recognize that he has reduced his intake of lactose or even milk products. If he says that he can reduce his diarrhea by altering his diet, find out specifically what he has eliminated and make up your own mind as to what he may in fact have done. In the case of steatorrhea a patient often fails to recognize that fat ingestion exacerbates the diarrhea and that the avoidance of fats ameliorates diarrhea. He may tell you only that he has found relief from a bland diet or a soft diet. Ask specifically what he means—ask about high-fat foods like gravy and fried foods.

Most patients with diarrhea have tried to take some medicine. The world is full of antidiarrheal agents. When such drugs seem to work well the cause is probably a toxic diarrhea, but in most other diarrheas they work poorly if at all. Patients often optimistically tell you that something-or-other helps, but if you press them you will usually not be convinced.

The widespread tendency of patients and physicians alike to treat diarrhea with such agents without investigation is unfortunate. The treatment of many remediable cases is delayed by such practices, sometimes fatally in the case of colonic carcinoma. The treatment of chronic diarrhea blindly with antidiarrheal agents is as illogical as treating a chronic fever with aspirin. Such agents mask (if only through a placebo effect) the symptoms of a particular pathologic process which itself must be discovered. The responsible process is not likely to be sought aggressively when the symptom is reduced or thought to be controlled.

Associated Symptoms in Diarrhea

Nausea and Vomiting

The sensation of nausea, with or without vomiting, generally accompanies distension of the hollow viscera. Accordingly nausea generally accompanies all high-volume diarrheas except colonic diarrheas. It is particularly severe in toxic diarrhea, where the mechanism of nausea may include some mechanism other than visceral distension; the responsible sensory nerve endings may be directly stimulated by bacterial toxins or the systemically absorbed toxins may produce direct excitation of the emetic centers in the brainstem. The resultant vomiting coupled with high-volume diarrhea can result in serious electrolyte and fluid depletion, far greater than in any other class of diarrhea except for the most extreme hormonal diarrhea.

Cramping Abdominal Pain

Cramps reflect the contraction of the intestinal muscle against an increased resistance. Both the resistance offered by the walls in partial mechanical obstruction and by the fluid load in high-volume diarrhea can produce cramps. Some degree of cramping characterizes many forms of diarrhea but severe cramping is especially characteristic of toxic diarrhea. Severe cramping also characterizes inflammatory obstruction of the terminal ileum, as occurs in Crohn's disease where the intensity of the pain often exceeds the intensity of the diarrhea.

The timing of cramps in relationship to defecation can suggest the source of the cramps. When the cramps mainly occur just before defecation, the source of cramping is most likely to be the colon and so you should suspect a form of colonic diarrhea. When the cramps are to some degree independent of defecation they more likely arise from the small intestine.

Altered Defecatory Sensation

The call to stool may be intensified in all forms of diarrhea. This intensification may involve the magnitude of the sensation, its tolerability and its frequency of recurrence if it is neglected. For these reasons this change in the call to stool is called *urgency,* and most patients know what you mean when you ask them about urgency to move the bowels. There is little to be gained from exploring the matter very far. Urgency seems to be mainly a function of the volume of the stool that is waiting to be delivered.

You should carefully distinguish between *urgency* and *tenesmus* because tenesmus has a very specific significance. Patients do not know the term, so you have to ask about it in the form of its definition. Tenesmus is an intense, often painful, urge to defecate, felt in the rectoanal region; it occurs frequently and is usually unproductive of anything except perhaps a small squirt of fluid or gas. It seems to represent the nearly continuous stimulation of the defecatory reflex by something other than normal mechanical stimulation of rectal mechanoreceptors. Tenesmus quite specifically accompanies proctitis of any cause and rectal neoplasm as well. The absence of tenesmus means nothing but its presence should point you to a colonic diarrhea in which the disease process involves the rectum.

Weight Loss

A tendency to lose weight accompanies all forms of diarrhea, obviously, since both water and calories are wasted. When a patient who complains of diarrhea denies weight loss I tend to assume that the diarrhea is functional or anxiety-related, and when weight loss has occurred I am likely to suspect that it is not. This is a common view held by physicians, but one of dubious validity, and I try to resist the tendency to think that way. People who are anxious may lose weight if they also suffer anorexia, and patients who have a small degree of caloric loss in the stool may successfully make it up by eating more.

The fact of weight loss alone is thus not particularly useful information but the rate and inexorability of weight loss are. You should be specific. Ask the patient what he weighed a week, a month or 6 months ago and what he weighs now. Ask him if he has tried to eat more to keep up. Continuous weight loss at a rate of 1 pound per week or more in the face of good caloric intake indicates loss of calories in the stool, and that points especially to malabsorptive and maldigestive diarrhea. When the diarrhea is associated with a neoplasm or a febrile illness, of course, weight loss may reflect these other processes as well. Where the diarrhea is more a loss of water than of calories, the weight loss is correspondingly more rapid. In either rapid or gradual weight loss, the weight falls more slowly as it approaches lean body mass. Thus in patients who have had depleting diarrhea for a very long time and who have become very malnourished, the weight tends to stabilize. Patients often interpret this as a good sign and they may not tell you, unless you ask, that they lost weight at first. You must therefore ask not only "Are you losing weight?" but also "Have you lost weight?"

Some patients never weigh themselves and they will say that they don't know if they have lost any. When you get such an answer, ask if the clothing is looser than it used to be. Don't assume that all patients are imaginative or observant enough to tell you this unless you ask.

A SUMMARY OF SOME FEATURES OF THE SIX CATEGORIES OF DIARRHEA

There are many things to ask about in the exploration of the specific features of a diarrheal illness. Some of these are very important and others less so. The most important features point you strongly in the right direction, the others are only suggestive. I have found six features to be most helpful in the categorization of diarrhea. Table 4-1 summarizes these six categories of diarrhea in terms of these six features. Even these six features are not equally important or reliable. They are listed in descending order of reliability from left to right. The presence of blood in the stool, a high stool volume, and a stool with a character that

Table 4-1. Six Categories of Diarrhea Interpreted in Terms of the Average Severity (− to +++) of Six Features of Diarrhea

	The Presence of Blood	High Stool Volume	Stool that Suggests Fat	Abruptness of Onset	Nausea and Vomiting	Cramping Pain
Ingestive diarrhea	−	+	−	+++ +++	−	−
Toxic diarrhea	++	+++	−	+++	+++	+++
Malabsorptive diarrhea	−	+++	+++	+ −	+ −	+ −
Maldigestive diarrhea	−	+	+++	+ −	+ −	+ −
Hormonal diarrhea	−	+++	−	+ −	+ −	+ −
Colonic diarrhea	+++	++	−	++	−	−

suggests a high fat content are all matters that patients are usually quite clear about and that you can easily verify at the bedside. The abruptness of onset, the intensity of nausea and vomiting, and the intensity of cramping pain are all more subjective matters. Thus one can use the first three features of diarrhea to construct a key to categorize diarrheas.

AN OUTLINE OR KEY TO FURTHER CATEGORIZE DIARRHEA

In this section I have used the three most reliable features of diarrhea (blood in the stool, stool volume, and fat in the stool) to present a scheme to arrive at the most common specific disease entities that can produce diarrhea. For such a purpose, the three main features must be considered as absolutes rather than as graded features; that is, all are to be regarded as present or absent rather than as present in various degrees. Under each of the categories of diarrhea, only the most common specific disease entities are listed. In this key, "grossly bloody stools" means a stool in which the blood is mixed with the stool; a "high stool volume" is more than an estimated 1 quart per day on the average; a "low stool volume" is less than an estimated 1 quart per day.

I. Grossly bloody stools
  A. High stool volume
    1. Colonic diarrhea
      a. Extensive ulcerative colitis
      b. Colitis due to colonic bacterial pathogens: *Shigella, Salmonella, Campylobacter, Clostridium difficile,* pathogenic *Escherichia coli.*
      c. Amebiasis, severe
  B. Low stool volume
    1. Colonic diarrhea
      a. Limited ulcerative colitis
      b. Limited colitis due to colonic bacterial pathogens: *Shigella, Salmonella, Campylobacter, Clostridium difficile,* pathogenic *E. coli*
      c. Crohn's disease of the colon
      d. Colonic carcinoma
      e. Diverticulitis

f. Ischemic colitis
g. Radiation colitis
h. Amebiasis, not severe

II. Fatty, foul, mushy, or sticky stools (Steatorrhea)
A. High stool volume
1. Malabsorptive diarrhea
a. Giardiasis
b. Celiac disease (nontropical sprue)
c. Intestinal bacterial overgrowth with nonpathogenic organisms
d. Postvagotomy diarrhea, severe
e. Extensive ileal resection (more than 100 cm)
f. Tropical sprue, severe
2. Maldigestive diarrhea
a. Pancreatic insufficiency, severe
B. Low stool volume
1. Malabsorptive diarrhea
a. Giardiasis, mild
b. Celiac disease (nontropical sprue), mild
c. Intestinal bacterial overgrowth with nonpathogenic organisms, mild
d. Postvagotomy diarrhea, mild
e. Extensive ileal resection (50 to 100 cm)
f. Tropical sprue, in the usual degree
2. Maldigestive diarrhea
a. Pancreatic insufficiency, in the usual degree

III. Watery stools (no blood, no features to indicate fat)
A. High stool volume
1. Toxic diarrhea
a. Enteritis or colitis due to infection with specific bacterial pathogens: *Shigella, Salmonella, Campylobacter, Clostridium difficile,* pathogenic *E. coli*
b. "Food poisoning"—ingestion of staphylococcal or clostridial toxins
c. Enterocolitis due to infection with various pathogenic viruses.
2. Hormonal diarrhea
a. Paraneoplastic diarrhea related most often to islet-cell tumors of the pancreas, medullary carcinoma of the thyroid, parathyroid adenoma, small-cell carcinoma of the lung, and malignant carcinoid
B. Low stool volume
1. Toxic diarrhea
a. All toxic diarrheas when they are ending (see III, A, 1, above)
2. Hormonal diarrhea
a. All hormonal diarrheas when they are beginning (see III, A, 2, above)
3. Ingestive diarrhea
a. Taking of magnesium-containing antacids
b. Surreptitious laxative use by the emotionally disturbed
c. Overindulgence in diet candies or foods containing sorbitol
d. Lactase or other disaccharidase deficiency

4. Colonic diarrhea
   a. All colonic diarrheas when they are mild (see I, B, 1, above)
   b. Functional or anxiety-related diarrhea

A DECISION WHEEL FOR DIARRHEA

Narrowing the list of causes for diarrhea requires consideration of a relatively few essential clinical features, though the minor features discussed in this chapter can also be useful in constructing a differential diagnosis. The essential features are the character of the stool and the stool volume. I have used these to prepare a decision wheel, diagrammed in Figure 4-1.

WHAT TO DO NEXT IN EXPLORING THE CAUSE OF DIARRHEA—SOME RULES

I did not intend that this book should include a full explanation of clinical diagnosis including laboratory investigations, but only that it should show how bedside logic can be used to point to the most direct and specific establishment of a diagnosis. With the symptom of diarrhea, almost more than with any other, such logic is important, for there are many causes of diarrhea and many ways to investigate it. A careful use of logic can spare patients a great deal in effort, money, discomfort, and time.

I have some rules that I find useful in this. These points may seem superfluous, but I have seen them all violated, to the disadvantage of patients.

Grossly bloody diarrhea nearly always arises from colonic disease. Therefore, if the stools are bloody start out by looking at the stool and the colon. Examine the stool to confirm that the color is really due to blood (and not overindulgence in beets, for example) by doing a guaiac or similar test. Look at some stool for pus cells and send it for culture for pathogens and for examination for ameba. Do this without a purge at first, then do a sigmoidoscopy to see if you can see mucosal inflammation. If you do, biopsy the mucosa. All this can be done at the first examination. If you have reason to suspect amebiasis then purge with sodium sulfate to obtain stool to examine. If this does not yield a diagnosis you will have to look at the whole colon. I prefer to do this first by colonoscopy rather than radiography because colonoscopy is much more revealing and specific.

Fatty stools nearly always come from either intestinal mucosal or pancreatic disease. You can strongly suspect steatorrhea from the clinical description and from the appearance and odor of the stool if you look at it and smell it, but you cannot be really sure. You can be convinced quickly if you do a Sudan stain. If this is negative you have not ruled out steatorrhea, but if it is positive you have ruled it in, unless the patient is taking mineral oil. This is very unlikely under the circumstances, but you should ask him. He may well deny it if he is an emotion-

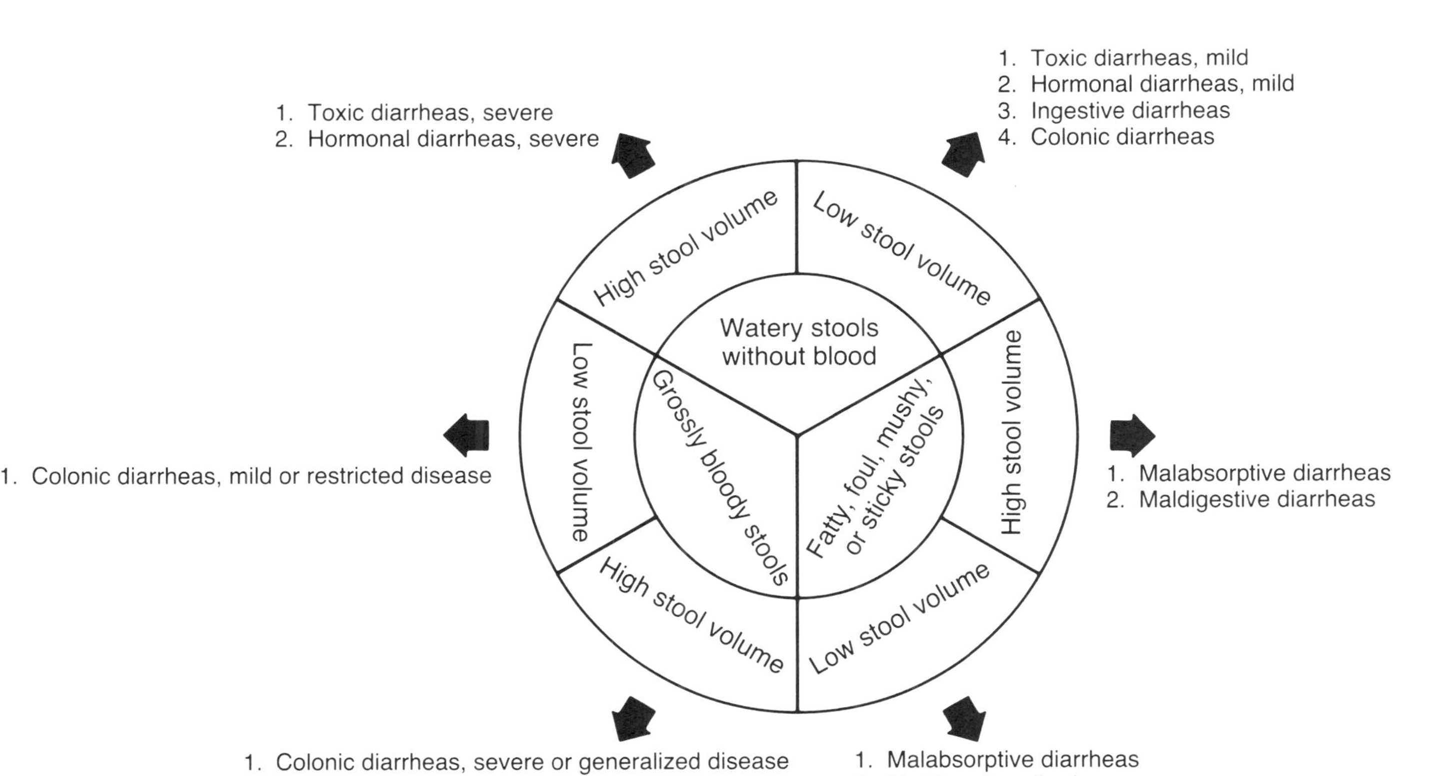

Fig. 4-1. A decision wheel classifying the general categories of causes of diarrhea on the basis of the character of the stool (core) and its estimated volume (periphery).

ally disturbed surreptitious taker of laxatives. When you are sure of steatorrhea, study the intestinal mucosa before the pancreas, unless you have strong reasons to suspect pancreatic insufficiency. The major intestinal causes of steatorrhea can be detected by histologic examination of the intestinal mucosa, examination of the duodenal aspirate for *Giardia,* and bacterial culture of the aspirate. You can do all these at one session, obtaining a duodenal biopsy with a peroral suction biopsy tube and a sample of duodenal contents through a duodenal tube for bacterial culture and microscopic examination for *Giardia.*

If the patient is "toxic" he probably has a toxic diarrhea. Since the majority of toxic diarrheas are due to infection of the gut lumen, you should culture the stool at the first examination, and then proceed according to the results.

If a watery diarrhea persists unchanged in volume during fasting, either he has a hormonal diarrhea or he is faking something. I am not completely certain of this rule. In most confirmed cases of hormonal diarrheas the stool volume is not much reduced in fasting, but I have seen and heard about patients with diarrhea who responded this way in whom an endocrine cause could not be established. That may only mean that there are diarrheogenic hormones yet to be discovered, but it could also be due to the Munchausen syndrome, in which smart and informed patients fake the signs of illness for their own private reasons. It is easy to produce fake diarrhea through the surreptitious ingestion of laxatives and the addition of water to the stool in the bedpan. It can be very difficult to rule out such practices, but convince yourself that you have before you proceed to look for hormonal causes of fasting-resistant watery diarrhea. When you embark on that course of laboratory investigation, you are heading into partially unknown territory where the goals can be elusive and expensive to reach. Remember that fasting-resistance in stool volume only means that enterocolonic mucosal secretion is a major mechanism in any case of diarrhea, and that it is one component of many causes for diarrhea where there is mucosal inflammation. In such cases fasting may reduce the volume somewhat, to the degree that mucosal secretion contributes to the volume of the stool.

It is easy to arrive too quickly at the diagnosis of "functional" or anxiety-related diarrhea, because you don't have to prove anything objectively. I do not deny that functional diarrhea exists, but it is clear that many diarrheal patients acquire this diagnosis incorrectly because of incomplete application of bedside observation and logic. Some quickly obtained evidence immediately points away from functional diarrhea—the presence of blood or fat in the stool, high stool volumes, and tenesmus, for example. But when such evidence is lacking, and more extensive logically applied investigations are fruitless, the possibility of functional diarrhea always arises. I keep two corollaries in mind in such a setting:

1. Anxiety-related diarrhea should not be my diagnosis unless I can find clear evidence of a *cause* for anxiety, and other evidence of the *effect* of anxiety. I usually ask a psychiatrist to help in this.
2. It is better for me to say "I don't know" and to be right, than it is for me to say "I know" and to be wrong.

5

CONSTIPATION AND RELATED SYMPTOMS: INCONTINENCE AND PAINFUL DEFECATION

WHAT DO PATIENTS MEAN WHEN THEY COMPLAIN OF CONSTIPATION?

Constipation is a lay term and it means somewhat different things to different people. The word mainly means a reduction in stool frequency, but it may also include the delivery of unusually hard or pelleted stools, painful defecation, the sensation of abdominal bloating, and abdominal cramping pain, separately or in various combinations; it may also encompass fecal incontinence, although that feature may not be volunteered by the constipated patient.

You cannot accept a complaint of constipation as the complete description of a symptom. Instead you must explore the exact nature of the problem. To do this you must use simple language, for few acceptable lay terms exist that can specifically identify the various features of constipation. You must use phrases like "the urge to move your bowels," "difficulty in making the stool pass," "pain when you pass a stool," "losing stool," and so on. Thus you can use simple and direct terms to discover exactly what patients mean when they say they are constipated. There are colloquial terms like "bound up," "plugged up," "corked," and so on that you will hear, and there are probably more, but they must vary with regions, they have variable shades of meaning and their use is unprofessional.

THE PHYSIOLOGY OF DEFECATION

Anal and Colonic Function in the Absence of Defecation

The structures of the rectum and anal canal and their nerves control defecation. In the resting state the striated muscles of the external anal sphincter and the pelvic floor are physiologically quite stable. They exhibit a constant low level of tone that can be raised by voluntary effort. The internal anal sphincter, a ring of smooth muscle that is continuous with the circular muscle layer of the rectum, differs from the rectal muscle in that it is tonically contracted to occlude the anal canal. The smooth muscle of the rectum itself is mostly flaccid but it exhibits intermittent weak contractions.

In the intervals between defecations, the rectum receives and holds the stool that descends from the distal colon. This descent seems quite slow normally; at least the sigmoidoscopist uncommonly finds very much stool there when he examines the unprepared patient. The temporal pattern of rectal filling is not clearly understood. Filling probably goes on intermittently over the long periods between defecations. It is widely accepted that the descent of stool into the rectum accelerates after eating. At least many people and animals defecate soon after eating a large meal. It is not clear whether this is a hormonally or neurally mediated effect.

The Preparatory Defecation Reflex

As the rectum fills it expands and elongates to accommodate the volume that it is receiving. This expansion continues until mechanoreceptive nerves somewhere in the rectal wall are excited by the distension of the rectal wall. It is not known exactly how these nerves are excited. They are mechanoreceptive, but it is not clear whether they are stretch-sensitive, pressure-sensitive, or movement-sensitive. The nerves responsible for the defecation reflex are thought to be the same as those responsible for the perception of the imminence of the reflex. They may be different in some way, though, because the perception can exist for a long time before the reflex is initiated.

The nerves to the rectum and anal canal are responsible for the coordination of events in defecation. The sensation of rectal fullness and the urge to defecate usually develop quite slowly. At some point the resting tone of the internal anal sphincter is inhibited as a part of the defecation reflex. This inhibition is accomplished by motor nerves that are neither adrenergic nor cholinergic (their transmitter is unknown) and the response is probably mediated in the distal spinal cord through pathways that traverse the pelvic nerves, pelvic plexus, and colonic nerves. The threat of untimely rectal evacuation when defecation is imminent can be overcome by voluntary contraction of the striated-muscle external anal sphincter. The urge to defecate usually fluctuates in intensity during the periods when defecation is resisted, but it is not clear that this fluctuation represents periodic rectal relaxations and contractions.

Events in Defecation

When the time comes to allow defecation to occur, a voluntary contraction of the abdominal wall muscles raises intra-abdominal pressure to force the rectal contents toward or into the anal canal. In some unknown way this intensifies the sensation of defecation and, from this point on, rectal evacuation becomes involuntary. Contraction of the rectal wall must occur during this event, but it is not known if it is peristaltic or simultaneous along the segment. The puborectalis contracts to pull the rectal apex anteriorly to straighten the segment, which presumably facilitates the completeness of its emptying. After rectal evacuation is complete the involved muscles return to their resting state.

SPECIFIC FEATURES OF CONSTIPATION

The Character of Constipation

Stool Frequency

In asking about frequency, first find out what the current situation of defecation is. Then ask about what the patient considers to be his normal stool frequency or stool "habit."

Patients who complain of constipation have infrequent stools, but the definition of abnormal stool frequency requires an idea of normal frequency. Normal people rarely talk about such a matter among themselves and physicians rarely ask patients with other complaints enough to discover what might be normal. From what I have read and found out by asking people, I accept three stools per week as the lower limit of normal. I consider two stools or less per week, on the average, as less than normal. A patient may consider two stools per week as severe constipation. It depends on what he has considered to be normal for him. Indeed, normal frequency is perhaps best defined on an individual basis. Some normal people have three stools daily for years on end and others three per week. Thus, a *change* in frequency is more significant than the absolute value.

Character of the Stool

Stool *consistency* in constipation is often changed so that stools are hard or contain hard segments. You should not assume that this is always so, for some constipated patients deliver stools of normal consistency. Sometimes a hard stool will be followed quickly by a formless stool.

Stool *color* may sometimes change in constipation. The normal brown color is normally intensified in a hard stool, but if the hard stool is very dark or black the patient is probably taking iron or bismuth, for both can cause constipation. In the black stool of melena the patient rarely complains of constipation, but you should always test a black stool for blood, even in constipation.

The Chronology of the Constipation

Onset

When you ask about the onset of constipation you will rarely get a very specific date, but occasionally you will. When the patient can be specific you should think of causes that might fairly abruptly obstruct the distal colon like carcinomas, postoperative strictures, or rapidly expanding inflammatory masses. In most causes of constipation, the onset is insidious.

Circumstances of Onset

If the patient can remember, even roughly, the period when the constipation began, ask him about other things that happened to him at that time. Did he change his diet or medications? Was he traveling? Did he change his level of physical activity? Did he have an abdominal operation? Some foods and many medicines produce constipation and the frequency of defecation seems to be greater in active people than in the sedentary. A period of enforced physical immobility, as occurs in a prolonged journey or in a period of convalescence from an illness, commonly produces constipation.

Periodicity

Like many chronic complaints constipation tends to recur periodically. When it does find out what circumstances seem to precipitate the episodes. When it is not a recurrent problem but a new and continuing (or progressing) episode you should think of obstructing lesions of the distal colon.

Progress

It is difficult to assess progression in constipation. Even when the complaint is constant and stable, constipation may seem to the patient to be getting worse simply because it does not go away. You can assess progression by asking about stool frequency, of course, but I find it much more useful to ask about the progress of treatments. Has the patient steadily increased his intake of laxatives? Has he progressed from glycerin suppositories through relatively mild laxatives like stool softeners, bulk-forming agents, and osmotics agents to more potent cathartics like phenolphthalein and bisacodyl to direct action with enemas? Is he now to the stage where he is trying anything and everything without much success? By asking about the progress of self-treatment you may get a graphic and convincing picture of progression. Steady progression signifies a progressive cause and suggests an increasing obstruction of the left colon.

Aggravating Factors in Constipation

Constipated patients usually think that certain things they eat make them worse. They either tell you about them or expect you to ask, but the information is not very helpful. A constipating diet will make constipation worse even if the main problem is an obstruction in the colon. The same is true for a sedentary life. To know that the constipation worsens when the patient is not getting much exercise is not much use. That happens in constipation of all causes.

Relieving Factors in Constipation

Most patients try diet changes, laxative drugs, and enemas seeking relief. Knowing what works is not very helpful in differential diagnosis. Neither is knowing what fails to work. Still, the patient expects you to ask what he has tried and this information can help you to judge progression and severity of the constipation, so you should explore relieving factors.

Associated Symptoms in Constipation

Blood with the Stool

When stools are very hard they may traumatize the anal canal to produce bleeding. This is especially likely to happen when hemorrhoids are present or when severe and prolonged straining at defecation distends the hemorrhoidal veins. You should ask about blood. If it is present ask especially about the relationship of bleeding to the passage of the stool. In hemorrhoidal bleeding the blood nearly always comes with the stool, being streaked on the surface of the stool, and it may continue to ooze from the anal canal for a moment or two after the stool has passed. Characteristically bright blood also appears on the toilet paper. If bleeding comes before the stool or is mixed with it, the bleeding site is somewhere above the anal canal.

Cramps and Bloating

Abdominal cramps and the sensation of bloating often accompany constipation. All causes of constipation can produce these symptoms, but they are most common and most severe in constipation due to a mechanical obstruction of the colon. Thus, you should try to assess their severity. Does the patient walk about holding his belly? Does the pain make him sweat? Does he have to loosen his clothing? If he does any of these things think of mechanical obstruction.

Nausea and Vomiting

Nausea is distinctly uncommon and rarely intense in constipation, and vomiting is rare. These symptoms, in general, arise because of distension of the hollow viscera, but the distension of the colon seems to be less capable of exciting nausea than distension of more proximal hollow organs. Even patients with nearly complete distal colonic obstruction from carcinoma do not often experience a major degree of nausea. For that reason, when nausea and vomiting are prominently associated with infrequent stooling you must strongly suspect an obstruction of the proximal colon or intestine, as in peritoneal adhesions, that is producing some degree of intestinal dilatation.

Incontinence of Stool

It may seem paradoxical to discuss incontinence in a discussion of constipation, but it is a frequent associated symptom and it is a significant one.

Incontinence arises because the mechanisms for continence fail. Continence is voluntary, and so it requires that the threat of the passage of stool is perceived and that the actions taken to achieve continence are effective. Thus continence can represent three things: failure of the stool to excite the signals for recognition, failure of the central nervous centers to recognize the signal, and failure of the normal voluntary motor efforts that bring about continence.

Excitation of the signal of recognition that stool is about to pass the anal canal seems to require a certain quantity and a certain solidity of the stool. Hence very liquid stools in small quantity are commonly not perceived and escape unnoticed. Any distal colonic obstruction, whether it is caused by a mass in the colonic wall or a hard mass of stool, is often bypassed by very liquid stool in small quantities from above, and so the patient may experience the unperceived passage of small liquid stools. Such incontinence does not necessarily imply a physiologic impairment of the defecation process.

When the incontinence is of larger quantities of formed stool, it signifies either defective generation of the signal of imminent stool passage or defective recognition of that signal. Defective signal generation is probably rare. It has not been investigated. Defective recognition of the signal is the best explanation for this form of incontinence, since it is common in patients with defective mentation of any cause and in patients with spinal cord injuries. Demented patients are often sedentary and sometimes receive constipating drugs (many psychotropic drugs are constipating), and so they may easily have constipation and incontinence of formed stool at the same time.

The inability of the patient to maintain continence when he knows he should signifies that the motor apparatus that he uses is somehow deranged. Because continence consists mainly in the voluntary contraction of the external anal sphincter and other striated muscles in the region, this form of incontinence can occur in many neuropathic and myopathic diseases. It is also a common consequence of trauma in the region, especially obstetric trauma to the external anal sphincter or pudendal nerves. When the perceived but uncontrollable passage of formed stool accompanies the complaint of constipation, the two complaints are probably related. For example many patients with neurologic and muscular diseases cannot bear down to defecate so they often develop constipation and they are sedentary. Yet they may develop incontinence of formed stool because of weakness of the pelvic floor muscles.

Weight Loss

Weight loss in association with constipation is very rare. In most causes of constipation, no loss of weight occurs because constipation does not importantly depress appetite, though patients may claim that it does. If you discover significant weight loss with constipation, especially if the constipation is a new and progressive complaint, you should suspect distal colonic cancer.

Painful Defecation (Dyschezia)

The passage of a hard stool often causes moderate pain in the anal canal. Constipated patients often assume that you know this so they may not mention dyschezia unless you ask about it. Dyschezia represents inflammation or cancer in the anal canal. You need to ask about the severity of dyschezia. The severity of the pain roughly parallels the depth of the disease process in the anal canal. If it has involved the anal sphincters, the pain is excruciating. When cancer of the anal canal causes dyschezia the dyschezia usually comes first, the constipation later.

Dyschezia can be both a consequence and a cause of constipation. It is a consequence when the repeated passage of very hard stools traumatizes the anal canal to set up a local inflammation. This may be only a mild cryptitis or papillitis, in which case the pain is mild; the inflammation may deepen to establish an anal fissure, which is very painful; if the fissure extends into the anal musculature, the pain is excruciating when a stool is passed, for the external sphincter is in reactive spasm and accepts dilatation only with considerable protest.

It is obvious why dyschezia can cause constipation. If defecation is an agony the victim will try hard not to defecate. Prolonged retention of the stool in the rectum and distal colon allows more water to be extracted from it so the stools become hard.

Thus, you must always explore dyschezia when it accompanies constipation. Is it only a little burning? Is it more than that? Is it agonizing? Find out if the pain developed first and the constipation afterward. This information can help you to anticipate what you find when you examine the anal canal in patients with dyschezia. When you do, proceed with special caution.

DISORDERS THAT CAUSE CONSTIPATION PRESENTED IN TERMS OF MECHANISMS

Most constipated patients can be classified into three reasonably distinct groups according to the major problem that seems to exist: those who have a deficient development of the urge to defecate (*colonic constipation*), those who sense the urge but cannot defecate (*somatomotor constipation*), and those who voluntarily suppress the urge because they have anal pain when they defecate (*dyschezic constipation*).

I have used these three categories to organize this presentation of specific clinical entities, and I have added two other categories, *truly massive constipation*, which calls to mind a special set of causes, and *endocrine constipation*.

You will find that many cases do not fall neatly into these categories. Also, some cases simply defy classification or explanation. This classification should, however, help you to think logically about the general topic of constipation and to deal with it sensibly.

Colonic Constipation

Most constipated patients will tell you that they rarely feel the urge to defecate. The problem may arise either because the rectum does not fill enough to excite the sensation or because the nerves that give rise to the sensation are defective. Both possibilities must exist, for some constipated patients are regularly found to have a filled rectum and others regularly found not to.

Defective Rectal Filling

Inadequate filling of the rectum can result from the impairment of colonic flow either because of depressed propulsive contractions of the colon, increased resistance to flow arising from the firmness of the fecal mass, or increased resistance to flow offered by an obstruction of the distal colonic wall. You should think of all three possibilities when you regularly encounter an empty rectum in a patient who says he is constipated and has not defecated just before you see him.

Of the three possibilities, it is widely believed that depressed colonic motility is the most common cause of such so-called simple constipation. An increased hardness of the fecal mass would be expected to result from prolonged retention of the stool and this hardness of the stool also impairs its movement. Thus the two processes, depressed colonic motility and fecal resistance to flow, are reinforcing. This probably explains why a short course of stool softeners or osmotic laxatives may end a period of constipation, permanently in some, but temporarily in others, for it breaks the cycle of reinforcement.

I presume the cycle can be initiated either by slowed colonic propulsion or by hard feces unusually resistant to forces impelling antegrade flow. The nature of the controls of colonic motility remains somewhat mysterious, but it seems likely that normal colonic motility is affected by many things. These could include physical activity and the emotional state as well as eating. At least it is a common observation that constipation often develops in circumstances of a sudden change in diet or reduction in physical activity (in traveling, for example), sharply reduced food intake, or depression. Of course depressed patients are often taking psychotropic drugs that are constipating, but constipation also occurs in those victims of depression who are not taking them. Psychotropic drugs probably initiate constipation by depressing colonic propulsive activity.

Certainly, unusually hard feces seem also sometimes to initiate constipation. I suppose very hard feces can occur with the ingestion of so-called constipating foods. Constipation due to hard feces is well known to occur in patients given suspensions of barium sulfate to drink in gastrointestinal radiography. Barium sulfate in suspension tends to form a very hard variably obstructing mass when it is dehydrated and this can be found to occur at any point along the colon. This may also be the reason for the well-known constipating effect of oral iron therapy.

You should not assume that "empty-rectum constipation" is always the result of depressed colonic motility or hard feces. Inadequate rectal filling is probably also the mechanism of the constipation complained of by those with occlusion of the distal colonic wall from cancer, inflammatory masses, and benign strictures.

Defective Rectal Sensation

When I find the rectum is regularly full of stool but no urge to defecate has occurred I assume that rectal sensation is faulty. This could possibly be due to sensory nerve disease confined to the anorectal area, but there is no way to establish that. It is more likely that it represents defective function of sensory spinal pathways or cerebral perception. Certainly "full-rectum constipation" is common in those who are demented or have spinal cord injury. This kind of constipation does not exclude colonic obstruction, from cancer for example, and you must not think that the finding of full-rectum constipation is reason to neglect a search for obstructing lesions.

Somatomotor Constipation

Somatomotor constipation is much more rare than colonic constipation. In somatomotor constipation the sensation seems to be normal but the victims cannot initiate or complete defecation because the required movements are not effectively accomplished. Because of the stool-filled rectum that is characteristically found in somatomotor constipation, you may confuse somatomotor constipation with the constipation of defective rectal sensation, but they can be distinguished if you convince yourself that the patient perceives the urge to defecate.

The first event in effecting defecation is the assumption of the appropriate posture for defecation; the second is the contraction of the abdominal wall musculature during suspension of respiration. The inability to complete either of these things impairs the voluntary advancement of the fecal mass into the distal rectum and anal canal. Such advancement can occur, of course, purely because of colorectal contractions, but often this is inadequate to maintain normal defecation. Defective somatomotor function is the mechanism of the constipation in patients who must remain supine, are fixed in body casts or frames, suffer from paraplegia or quadriplegia, have pain with abdominal wall contraction (as after abdominal operations), have such severe pulmonary insufficiency that they cannot suspend respiration, or suffer striated-muscle weakness from primary muscle disease.

Dyschezic Constipation

Dyschezia can readily cause constipation because the patient finds it painful to defecate. The various degrees of inflammatory disease of the anal canal all can cause constipation. These include cryptitis, papillitis, fissures, and pararectal abscesses. Squamous-cell carcinoma of the anus can produce dyschezia as well. The healing of anorectal inflammation or the incision of a hemorrhoidectomy may cause a residual anal stricture and that can cause dyschezic constipation too.

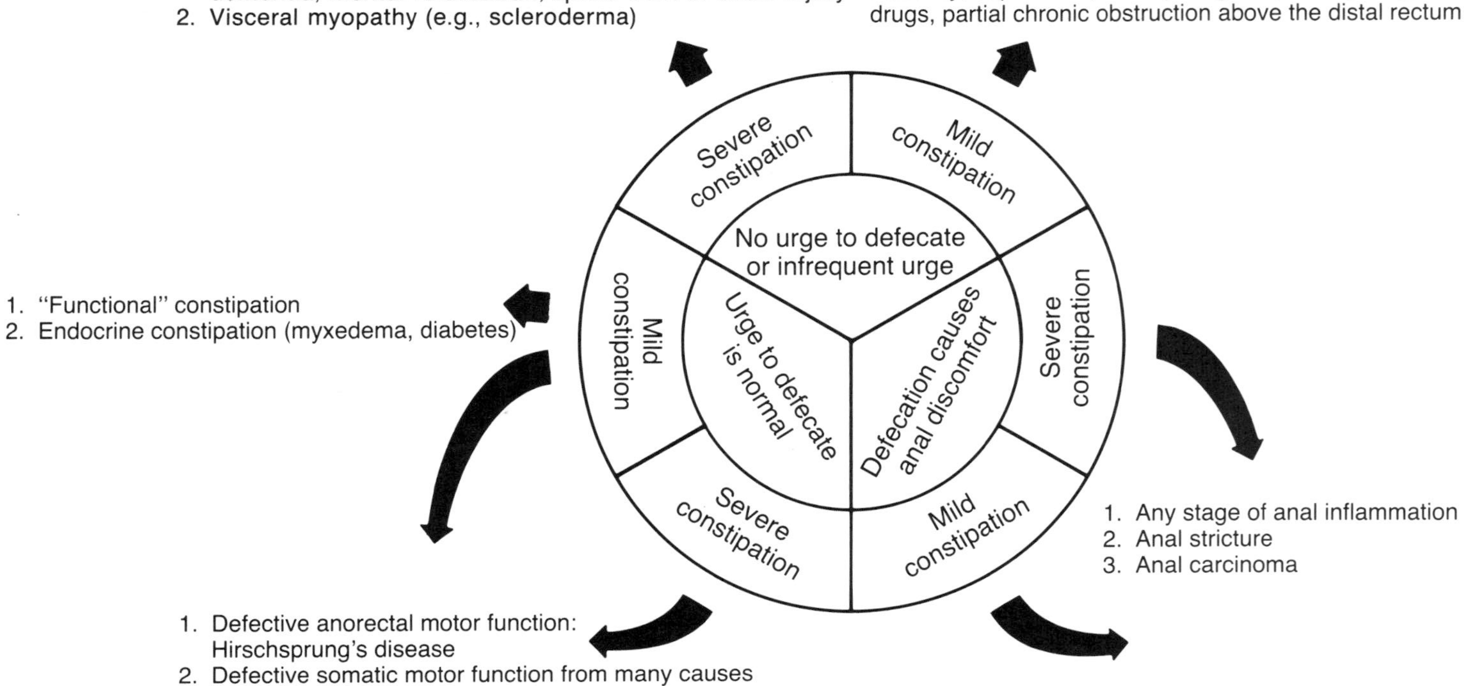

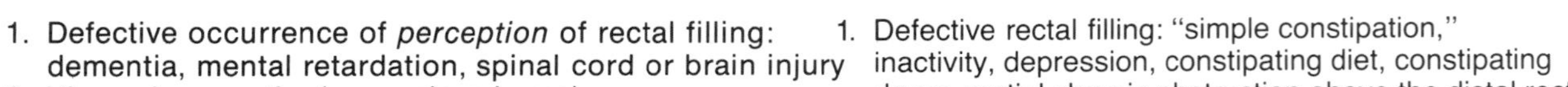

Fig. 5-1. A decision wheel classifying the causes of constipation on the basis of the nature of the urge to defecate (core) and the degree of constipation (periphery).

Truly Massive Constipation

Most of the causes of constipation briefly presented in the preceding categories produce a degree of constipation that may seem quite severe, but it is mild compared to that which can occur in a few situations. The category of truly massive constipation should occur to you when you find an appropriate history, evident abdominal distension, and massive dilatation and elongation of the colon. Of course, some of the forms of colonic, somatomotor, or dyschezic constipation can create these findings if the causes have been present for a very long time.

Truly massive constipation is often found in patients with long-standing defective mentation, especially in those with congenital mental retardation. In such cases the constipation may have begun as defective rectal sensation aggravated by fecal impaction. Such patients also typically have received large doses of psychotropic drugs and laxatives. Chronic laxative use is always associated with chronic constipation and some people believe that certain laxatives taken chronically impair colonic motor function—that the cure contributes to the cause.

Disorders that cause fibrosis in visceral smooth muscle can cause truly massive constipation. The common one is diffuse systemic sclerosis or scleroderma. The other collagen diseases rather rarely do so. The primary visceral myopathies, recently described, also can cause truly massive constipation.

Endocrine Constipation

Constipation is common in hypothyroidism. The mechanisms involved are not clear. Chronic constipation is said to be the most common gastrointestinal complaint of patients with diabetes mellitus, but this is thought to be a manifestation of autonomic neuropathy.

A DECISION WHEEL FOR CONSTIPATION

Narrowing the list of causes in any case of constipation requires the consideration of relatively few essential features. The most useful are the sensory features (presence or absence of the urge to defecate the painful defecation) and the estimated severity of the problem. The use of these features is diagrammed in Figure 5-1.

6

JAUNDICE

THE DEFINITION OF JAUNDICE

What Patients Call Jaundice

Jaundice means simply a yellow complexion. By convention we use the term to refer to the color of the skin produced by the accumulation of bilirubin in the tissues, but a similar color occurs in the skin of people who consume large amounts of carotene-containing vegetables or take quinacrine chronically. Some jaundiced patients may complain only of yellow eyes because they notice the color there. Others may describe the complexion as pale, or only as being changed in some way.

"Jaundice is the disease your friends diagnose," said Osler. The color is obscured by the yellow light of incandescent lamps so patients often miss it since they look at themselves mostly in the early morning and evening. Other people see them more in the sunlight when jaundice is easier to detect. Some causes of jaundice also cause generalized itching or dark urine and some patients will notice first the itching that sometimes accompanies jaundice or the dark urine before they observe the jaundice itself.

What You Should Look For

Jaundice is both a complaint and a physical finding, so you should inspect the skin carefully when a patient says that he is jaundiced. You can easily do some of this inspection as he is talking and you should do the rest in the physical examination. There are a few simple points to remember.

You should use natural light, the brighter the better, for jaundice is very hard to see in artificial light, especially fluorescent light. Slight degrees of jaundice can be hard to see. It is helpful to look at someone else of similar complexion in the same light at the same time.

Bilirubin in the skin is easily obscured by melanin. It is easier to see jaundice in areas of skin not commonly exposed to the sun, the skin of the abdomen, palms, and soles, so you should look critically at these areas. In blacks and other dark people you can best see jaundice in the sclerae and under the tongue. You must look at the sclerae in all cases, though, to confirm that the jaundice is really that. Yellowing of the skin without yellowing of the sclerae indicates hypercarotenemia. The yellow vegetable pigment, carotene, is fat-soluble so it is not concentrated in fat-poor tissues like the sclerae, while bilirubin is distributed everywhere. In dark people and people who are "weathered" from prolonged outdoor exposure the sclerae often contains some melanin pigment peripherally so you should focus on the sclera around the limbus in looking for jaundice.

Look for excoriations in the skin in regions accessible to scratching, like the forearms and abdomen. Excoriations indicate that itching is severe and supports the idea that any detectable yellowness of the skin is due to bilirubin accumulation. When you see excoriations ask if the itching is a generalized pruritus or if it is localized, suggesting a local lesion. Itching in jaundice is usually generalized. It is sometimes most intense in the palms and soles.

WHAT YOU NEED TO KNOW ABOUT BILIRUBIN METABOLISM TO INTERPRET JAUNDICE AT THE BEDSIDE

Bilirubin metabolism is very complicated and hard to remember. In the application of bedside logic you need only to remember it as a series of four steps: the production of bilirubin from hemoglobin, the uptake and conjugation of bilirubin by hepatocytes, the excretion of conjugated bilirubin from hepatocytes into bile canaliculi, and the transit of conjugated bilirubin as bile flows along the biliary tree.

The Production of Bilirubin from Hemoglobin

Most of the bilirubin excreted by the liver comes from the enzymatic degradation of hemoglobin from red cells. A little comes from other sources. Reticuloendothelial cells of the marrow, spleen, and liver remove aged and damaged red cells from the circulation, destroy them, and degrade the liberated hemoglobin to bilirubin. This bilirubin enters the plasma where it is bound to albumin.

The Uptake and Conjugation of Bilirubin by Hepatocytes

Hepatocytes dissociate plasma bilirubin from albumin and take it up rapidly by a carrier-mediated process. The bilirubin is enzymatically conjugated to glucuronic acid allowing it to be excreted in the bile.

The Excretion of Bilirubin into Bile Canaliculi

Hepatocytes excrete the conjugated bilirubin into the bile canaliculi through another carrier-mediated process. This is the slowest event in the sequence of steps: it is the rate-limiting step in bilirubin metabolism.

The Transit of Bilirubin along the Biliary Tree

Under the low pressure of bile secretion bile flows continuously along converging canaliculi, ductules and ducts. About 60 percent of the bile enters the gallbladder while about 40 percent flows directly to the duodenum. The sphincter of Oddi acts as a peristaltic pump rather than as a regulating valve. Bile that enters the gallbladder is concentrated there. It is periodically expelled into the duodenum as the gallbladder contracts in response to eating.

HOW JAUNDICE COMES ABOUT

Bilirubin accumulates in the body when the excretion of bilirubin in the bile cannot keep up with production. Thus jaundice can represent either overproduction of bilirubin or defective operation of the uptake-conjugation, excretion, or transit steps.

These steps take place in different organs. The production of bilirubin occurs mainly in places remote from the liver, abdomen, and gastrointestinal tract; uptake-conjugation and excretion occur in the liver; transit occurs below the liver, in the biliary tree. Bilirubin that has not been conjugated may accumulate, waiting to be taken up by hepatocytes. Bilirubin that has been conjugated may also accumulate in the blood by diffusing back into the blood because something is blocking its excretion or transit.

A SIMPLE CLASSIFICATION OF THE CAUSES OF JAUNDICE

There are several ways to classify the causes of jaundice. The simple classification given here can help you arrive at probable causes with some precision through the application of logic at the bedside. To designate the five categories listed, I use some unconventional terms because I find them more useful than the conventional terms, which are supplied in parentheses.

- Jaundice that is *not* due to intra-abdominal disease
  - Overproduction jaundice (*hemolytic jaundice*)
  - Eponymic jaundice (*congenital jaundice*), due to a congenital enzymatic defect in bilirubin handling
- Jaundice that *is* due to intra-abdominal disease
  - Uptake-conjugation jaundice (*hepatocellular jaundice*), due to diffuse damage to hepatocytes
  - Excretory jaundice (*cholestatic jaundice*), due to a deficit in hepatocyte excretory function
  - Obstructive jaundice, due to obstruction of the flow of bile in the biliary tree

In this classification you should think of overproduction jaundice or eponymic jaundice when none of the information you receive at the bedside suggests intra-abdominal disease. When the information does suggest intra-abdominal disease, you must decide which of the three forms listed above is favored. Uptake-conjugation and excretion take place inside the liver. If you interpret other bedside information as indicating the presence of disease of the liver, that favors defective uptake-conjugation or excretion. Transit takes place outside the liver. If other information indicates disease of other abdominal organs than the liver, that favors defective transit or obstructive jaundice.

A FULLER EXPLANATION OF THE FIVE CLASSES OF JAUNDICE

Overproduction Jaundice

I call this an *overproduction jaundice* rather than hemolytic jaundice because the term *hemolysis* is commonly used to mean only intravascular hemolysis, and this usage excludes the destruction of red cells in hematomas and purpura. Excessive production of bilirubin from degradation of hemoglobin can come about by both intravascular and extravascular hemolysis, and it occurs in ineffective hematopoiesis. This category includes all those situations in which excess bilirubin is delivered to the liver. Overproduction is not often the sole cause of jaundice, since the capacity of the liver to remove bilirubin greatly exceeds the normal rate of bilirubin production. What appears to be overproduction is generally overproduction combined with mildly defective hepatic bilirubin excretion. The hepatic excretory defect is mild, stable, and unsuspected until the system is stressed by the presentation of a large load of bilirubin from a bout of intravascular hemolysis or an extensive interstitial hemorrhage. The important point is that, even when an episode of jaundice seems to you to be hemolytic, you should not fail to consider other defects in bilirubin metabolism too. Some of the common diseases that cause overproduction jaundice are listed in Table 6-1.

Eponymic Jaundice

I call this *eponymic jaundice* rather than congenital jaundice, because all forms of congenital jaundice are nearly universally referred to by their eponyms rather than by their descriptive names. This eponymic terminology makes it difficult for the nonhepatologist to remember what the exact metabolic defects are. On the other hand, the descriptive names are so long, so complicated, and so similar that I have trouble remembering them. If it were not for the fact that Gilbert's syndrome is so common, it would not matter a great deal, since the other forms of eponymic jaundice are so rare as to be of less than major practical importance.

These forms of jaundice are all due to congenital enzymatic defects that interfere with the uptake, conjugation, or excretion of bilirubin by the hepatocytes. None of them is actually a form of liver disease, since the liver works well in

Table 6-1. Conditions Exemplifying the Five Clinical Classes of Jaundice

Overproduction jaundice
- Intravascular hemolysis, including ineffective hematopoiesis
- Extravascular hemolysis from hematomas
- Competitive binding to albumin by certain drugs

Eponymic jaundice
- Gilbert's syndrome (idiopathic unconjugated hyperbilirubinemia)
- Crigler-Najjar syndrome (congenital nonhemolytic jaundice)
- Dubin-Johnson syndrome (chronic idiopathic jaundice)
- Rotor's syndrome (familial chronic conjugated hyperbilirubinemia)

Uptake-conjugation jaundice
- Diffuse hepatocellular disease
  - Hepatitis due to infectious agents
  - Hepatocellular toxicity from alcohol, drugs and other toxins
- Diffuse infiltrative disease of the liver
  - Malignant infiltrations, like carcinomas and lymphomas
  - Benign infiltrations, like sarcoidosis, amyloidosis, hemochromatosis

Excretory jaundice
- Drugs that interfere with bilirubin secretion, like 17-alpha alkylated steroids
- Drugs that impair intrahepatic bile flow, like estrogen and phenothiazines
- Diseases of intrahepatic biliary radicals, like pericholangitis and primary biliary cirrhosis

Obstructive jaundice
- Intraductal disease, like stones, strictures, sclerosing cholangitis, and cholangiocarcinoma
- Extraductal disease, like pancreatic edema, pancreatic carcinoma, and malignant or inflammatory lymph nodes at the porta hepatis

most other respects. The jaundice in Gilbert's syndrome is in part an example of overproduction jaundice, since the jaundice characteristically only appears after an episode of physical stress, like an injury, a surgical operation, a febrile illness, or a period of fasting. In some such stresses, hemolysis may be increased and it is possible that this transient overproduction, added to the minor defect in hepatic bilirubin metabolism, is what causes the mild jaundice that characterizes Gilbert's syndrome. The forms of eponymic or congenital jaundice are summarized in Table 6-1.

Uptake-Conjugation Jaundice

I call this *uptake-conjugation jaundice* rather than hepatocellular jaundice because that term says what hepatocellular processes are defective. Hepatocellular jaundice should strictly include all causes of jaundice due to any dysfunction of hepatocytes. Because the excretion of conjugated bilirubin into the canaliculi is one such hepatocyte function, the term hepatocellular jaundice should logically include the distinct form of jaundice called intrahepatic cholestasis (due to defective bilirubin excretion), but the term is not used that way. The distinction is important, since uptake-conjugation jaundice is commonly associated with a general disturbance of hepatocyte function and structure while intrahepatic cholestasis (defective bilirubin excretion) is often not. The causes and implications of uptake-conjugation jaundice and intrahepatic cholestasis (excretory jaundice) are rather different.

There are three categories of uptake-conjugation jaundice: that associated with *acute inflammation* of the liver from infectious agents or drugs; that associated with *chronic inflammation* of the liver, most forms of which are sometimes accompanied by cirrhosis; and that associated with *infiltrative diseases* of the liver, both malignant and benign. The latter causes may produce jaundice in part because of obstruction to bile flow, but they also may impair hepatocyte function because they interfere with the delivery of bilirubin, or they may impede hepatic blood flow or damage hepatocytes directly. The most common specific entities in these three categories are summarized in Table 6-1. Because many hepatocyte functions besides bilirubin uptake and conjugation are defective in hepatocellular jaundice, the causes of jaundice in this category are frequently characterized by other signs of liver disease.

Excretory Jaundice

I call this *excretory jaundice* rather than cholestatic jaundice because that tells me what process is defective. *Cholestasis* (stasis of bile) could refer to obstruction of the bile ducts; indeed, the term is sometimes used that way by those who refer to mechanical bile duct obstruction as "extrahepatic cholestasis" and the intrahepatic physiologic abnormality as "intrahepatic cholestasis"; in fact the former is a problem of obstruction and the latter a problem of defective production and intrahepatic flow of bile. Excretory jaundice is due to a defect in the operation of two steps in the handling of bilirubin: the excretion of conjugated bilirubin from the hepatocytes and the flow of bile in canaliculi and ductules. Defective excretion can occur as a part or stage of uptake-conjugation jaundice of any kind, but it often appears to be the major perceptible defect, especially in drug-induced jaundice. Some drugs in current use that can cause excretory jaundice with an incidence of more than about 1 percent appear in Table 6-2.

Obstructive Jaundice

Obstruction to the flow of bile through the extrahepatic ducts produces jaundice because the conjugated bilirubin diffuses from the bile, backed up above the obstruction, through the liver, and into the bloodstream. Very little diffusion occurs through the epithelium of the biliary tract. The degree of jaundice reflects the degree of obstruction. Obstructive jaundice is usually caused by one of two things: stones in the ducts or compression of the distal duct by the head of the pancreas through which it passes. Obstruction by the pancreas arises either from inflammation or neoplasm. Intrinsic lesions of the bile duct (strictures, sclerosing cholangitis, cholangiocarcinoma) are less common. Occasionally, extrinsic tumors like tumor-laden nodes at the porta hepatis cause obstructive jaundice. Some causes of obstructive jaundice are listed in Table 6-1.

Table 6-2. Some Common Drugs in Current General Use Reported to Cause Jaundice with Appreciable Frequency by Cholestasis (Ch) and by Hepatocellular Injury (H)

Agent	Mechanism
I. Anesthetics	H
A. Halothane	
B. Methoxyflurane	
C. Fluoroxene	
II. Psychotropics and anticonvulsants	
A. Tranquilizers	
1. Phenothiazines	Ch
Chlorpromazine	
Fluphenazine	
Mepazine	
Thioridazine	
Triflupromazine	
2. Thioxanthines	Ch
Chlorprothixene	
Clopenthixol	
Thiothixene	
3. Butyrophenones	Ch
Haloperidol	
4. Benzodiazepines	Ch
Chlordiazepoxide	
Diazepam	
B. Antidepressants	
1. Hydrazines	H
Isocarboxazid	
Nialamide	
Pheniprazine	
Phenoxypropazine	
2. Tricyclic antidepressants	Ch
Amitriptyline	
Desipramine	
Doxepin	
Imipramine	
Nortriptyline	
Protriptyline	
C. Anticonvulsants	H
Diphenylhydantoin	
Mephenytoin	
Paramethadione	
Trimethadione	
III. Antirheumatic agents	H or Ch
Acetaminophen	
Phenylbutazone and derivatives	
Dantrolene	
IV. Hormone derivatives and drugs used to treat endocrine disease	
A. Steroids	Ch and H
Anabolic (C-17 alkylated) steroids	
Estrogenic hormones and related drugs	
Oral contraceptives	
B. Oral hypoglycemics	Ch
Chlorpropamide	
C. Antithyroid drugs	H or Ch
Propylthiouracil	
Methimazole	

(*Table continues.*)

Table 6-2. Continued

Agent	Mechanism
V. Antimicrobials and antiparasitic agents	
A. Antibiotics	
Clindamycin	H
Erythromycin estolate	Ch
Carbenicillin	H
Oxacillin	H
Tetracycline (large IV dosage)	H
Triacetyloleandomycin	H and Ch
B. Synthetic antimicrobials	
Sulfonamides	H
Sulfones	H and Ch
Arsenicals	H and Ch
Nitrofurantoin	H and Ch
C. Antiprotozoal agents	
Antimonials	H
D. Antituberculous agents	
Isoniazid	H
Ethionamide	H
Pyrazinamide	H
Para-amino salicylic acid	H
Rifamycin	H
VI. Drugs used to treat cardiovascular disease	
A. Antiarrhythmic agents	
Quinidine	H
B. Antihypertensive agents	
Alpha-methyldopa	H
C. Drugs used to treat hypercholesterolemia	
Nicotinic Acid	Ch
D. Anticoagulants	
Phenindione	H
VII. Antineoplastic agents	H
A. Antimetabolites	
Methotrexate	
6-Mercaptopurine	
Antipyridimines	
Asparaginase	
Mithramycin	
Puromycin	
VIII. Other drugs	
Acetaminophen	H

OVERLAPS IN THE CAUSES OF JAUNDICE

The mechanisms of jaundice do not often operate alone in any single case except for excretory and obstructive jaundice. In most cases one can see some evidence for two or more causes working at the same time. Thus, for example, in the jaundice due to Gilbert's syndrome both the congenital enzymatic defect and overproduction of bilirubin may be present. In hepatocellular jaundice both uptake-conjugation and excretion are defective. There is great risk in identifying causes of jaundice only in terms of one mechanism, for you may miss other disease by doing so. You must, therefore, keep all mechanisms in mind as you evaluate a patient with jaundice. If you always consider the four processes systematically in descending order along the pathway—production, uptake-conjugation, excretion, and transit—you will not miss thinking of them all.

THE SPECIFIC FEATURES OF JAUNDICE

The Character of Jaundice

Jaundice is usually a fairly bright yellow color, but some patients may see it as greenish or brownish, and you may too. Such color shift only means that the jaundice has been present for a long time. It may be due to chemical changes in the bilirubin in the skin with time or light-exposure or to secondary stimulation of melanin production.

The Location of Jaundice

Jaundiced patients often complain that their eyes are most affected when the eyes are really only most conspicuously affected. Bilirubin is distributed uniformly in all body tissues in jaundice. It is clearest in those regions that are relatively free of melanin: the palms, soles, abdominal skin, and bottom of the tongue.

The Chronology of Jaundice

Onset

The onset of jaundice is usually described as fairly abrupt, since patients know it is abnormal and seek help immediately when they detect it. Usually they do not observe it until the hyperbilirubinemia has been present for some time. Thus knowing the nature of the onset is not helpful.

Progression

The progression of jaundice is also not very useful information. The severity of jaundice does not fluctuate from day to day, even when the serum bilirubin fluctuates, because the tissues constitute a large reservoir to which bilirubin has access only by diffusion from plasma. The slowness of such diffusion allows skin color to follow changes in plasma bilirubin concentrations only after several days. Patients often tell you that jaundice fluctuates from day to day, but this is the result of wishful thinking and the vagaries of the intensity of daylight.

Circumstances of Onset

The circumstances of onset are very important to find out about, since jaundice is often due to the effects of drugs or chemicals on the liver. You must ask if patients are taking any of the recognized hemolytic or hepatotoxic drugs and you must be very specific. Do not simply ask the patient if he has been taking any drugs. Ask him to identify them and to tell you why he was taking the medicine. He may need to show you the bottle, to describe the pills (color, shape, size, surface markings), or, if these fail, to pick them out of a page of colored pictures of pills like that you find in the *Physician's Desk Reference.* Note all the drugs he is taking. Some, like chlorpromazine, are famous and frequent hepatotoxins, while others are less obvious. You must ask about exposure to many industrial chemicals that are hemolytic or hepatotoxic, at work and at home. People these days are generally more aware of environmental chemicals as causes of jaundice than they are of drugs so it is usually easier to find out about chemicals than it is about drugs in talking about the circumstances of the onset. You must be as persistent in inquiring about chemicals as you are in reviewing drugs. Be sure to ask about alcohol and do not forget suicide attempts.

Previous Episodes

You must ask about previous episodes of jaundice. Some diseases that cause jaundice are diseases that show exacerbations and remissions, and so a history of previous episodes of jaundice can suggest such a disorder. When exposure to drugs or chemicals is clearly related to the onset of jaundice, the jaundice is most likely to be due either to defective uptake-conjugation or to defective excretion. Drugs and chemical agents can produce jaundice both by damaging the hepatocytes to produce uptake-conjugation jaundice and by selectively depressing hepatocyte excretion of conjugated bilirubin, excretory jaundice. It is also possible that such an association could suggest hemolytic jaundice, since some patients develop mild hemolysis when they take certain drugs. This is unlikely because the capacity of the normal liver to excrete bilirubin is hardly ever exceeded except in extreme degrees of hemolysis.

Aggravating Factors in Jaundice

Aggravating factors, if commented on at all, are usually imaginary and the information is generally useless. The main exception is the jaundice of Gilbert's syndrome in which patients may notice that jaundice occurs with physical stress, fasting, or minor febrile illnesses. Jaundiced patients will often say that the jaundice seems to worsen with fatigue or at the end of the day.

Relieving Factors in Jaundice

Relieving factors, if commented upon at all, are imaginary and the information is useless. Jaundiced patients often say that the jaundice gets better with rest.

Associated Symptoms in Jaundice

The associated symptoms are the most important features that allow you to categorize jaundice at the bedside. Such an association often is not evident to a patient. The associated symptoms are often perceived as being unrelated to the jaundice. For this reason you must ask about each associated symptom specifically, asking if it was noticed either before or since the jaundice was first noticed. The most important associated symptoms are abdominal pain, nausea and vomiting, itching, and bloating.

Abdominal Pain

The occurrence of any kind of abdominal pain with jaundice suggests strongly that the jaundice is due to intra-abdominal disease. The conclusion is made even stronger if the nature of the abdominal pain suggests that the liver, biliary tract, or pancreas is the source. The *location* of pain is the most useful indicator of the organ or origin. Liver pain is maximal over the area of the liver in the right upper quadrant and may extend into the chest. Biliary tract pain is usually more caudad in the right upper quadrant and it may radiate to the right intrascapular area. Pancreatic pain is epigastric or periumbilical in its primary location. It often projects through to the back in the midline lumbar area where it may be as intense as it is anteriorly. If the nature of the pain strongly suggests the biliary tract or the pancreas as its source, then the associated jaundice is most likely to be obstructive jaundice. Obstructions most often arise from the biliary tract in the form of stones and from the pancreas in the form of cancer or pancreatitis. If the nature of the pain is such that the liver seems to be the origin, then the jaundice is likely to be due either to defective uptake-conjugation or to defective excretion of bilirubin. If the abdominal pain suggests some other organ, you cannot firmly classify the jaundice on that basis. For example, even if the pain arises from a malignancy (of the stomach or colon, for example), the jaundice could be obstructive because of obstruction of the hepatic ducts, or it could be due to defective hepatocyte function because of diffuse hepatic metastasis.

Nausea and Vomiting

Like abdominal pain, nausea in association with jaundice almost always means that the jaundice is due to intra-abdominal disease. Nausea and vomiting are especially prominent with abdominal diseases in which a hollow viscus is distended rapidly by a high-grade obstruction, or in which a solid organ enlarges so rapidly as to stretch its capsule. Thus nausea and vomiting are suggestive of obstructive jaundice (in which the biliary tree and gallbladder are distended) but only when the obstruction is sudden, acute, and relatively high-grade, as occurs in gallstones; when the obstruction is insidious, slow, and incomplete, as occurs in pancreatic carcinoma, nausea and vomiting are not often so prominent. Nausea and vomiting are also prominent when the liver itself enlarges rapidly, but not when it enlarges slowly. Thus nausea is common with the jaundice of hepatitis, where the liver swells rapidly, but not in alcoholic cirrhosis, where the liver enlarges slowly.

Itching

Generalized itching associated with jaundice always means that the jaundice represents intra-abdominal disease. Such itching feels deep in the skin and is poorly relieved by scratching. Itching in jaundice represents the action on the skin of some substance, possibly a bile salt, that hepatocytes excrete into the bile along with conjugated bilirubin. Thus itching is a reliable indicator of either obstructive or excretory jaundice. Obstructive jaundice is almost always due to gallstones, pancreatic cancer, or inflammation, while defective excretion of bile is most often due to drugs. The itching does not parallel the jaundice in severity. It is present only in about two-thirds of cases of obstructive jaundice and in a smaller proportion of cases of excretory jaundice. Thus its absence has little meaning in the interpretation of jaundice.

Bloating

A sensation of bloating in association with jaundice nearly always means that the jaundice arises from intra-abdominal disease. It can tell you little more, however, for this sensation accompanies a great many causes of jaundice.

General or Systemic Complaints

Such complaints as fatigue, an increased sleep requirement, or diminished tolerance for exertion are all useful to ask about. These may accompany many diseases characterized by jaundice, but they are especially characteristic of acute viral hepatitis where they may begin many days before the jaundice appears. This is true also of alterations in the sense of taste of foods and tobacco. These changes may make patients stop eating and smoking well before the onset of jaundice.

SOME NONABDOMINAL PHYSICAL SIGNS THAT MAY ACCOMPANY JAUNDICE

Certain nonabdominal physical signs are sometimes considered useful clues to the existence of chronic liver disease as the cause of jaundice. Indeed, they may be, but they are not very dependable.

Vascular Spiders

These lesions, well-described in many textbooks of physical diagnosis, are clearly related to chronic alcoholic liver disease. The problems in dealing with this physical sign are (1) confusing spiders with telangiectasias and (2) knowing

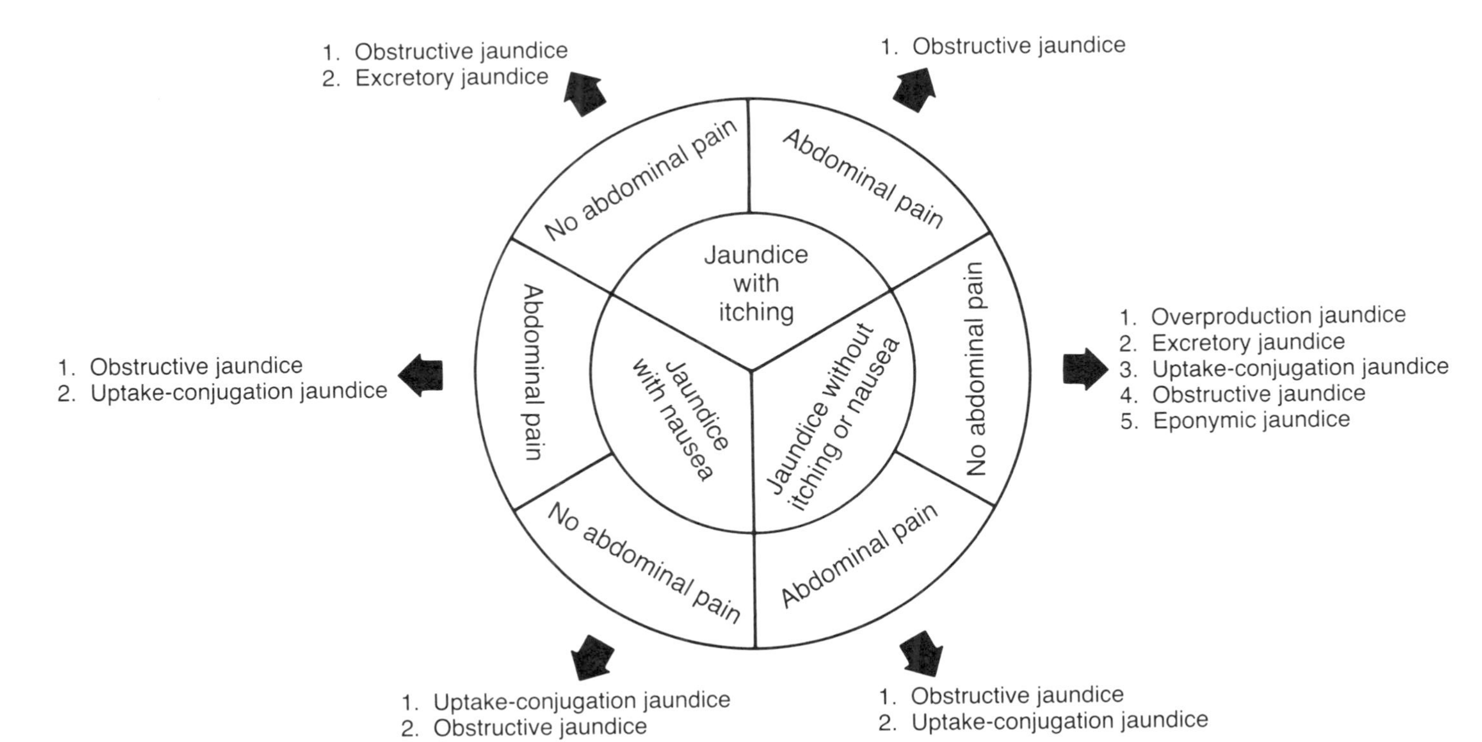

Fig. 6-1. A decision wheel classifying the general categories of the causes of jaundice on the basis of the presence of associated symptoms.

how many spiders normal people have. As for the former problem, it is easy to demonstrate the characteristic filling from the central vessel in a spider by compressing it with your fingertip or a glass microscope slide to empty the spider and then watching it fill. You should do that in suspect lesions before you count them as spiders. As for the latter problem, an authority on spiders has told me that a normal man can have up to a total of three spiders, a normal woman up to nine. Spiders, both normal and pathologic, are usually above the nipple line, but no one knows why this is so. An increased number of vascular spiders is more strongly suggestive of alcoholic liver disease than of other kinds.

Palmar Erythema

Though often taken as evidence of chronic liver disease, palmar erythema is not a reliable sign. Some healthy people have it and many victims of alcoholic liver disease do not.

Contracture of the Palmar Fascia

Contracture of the palmar fascia, like palmar erythema, is often cited as a sign of chronic liver disease. With a lesion that is so common as this one is in healthy people, such an association cannot easily be proved.

Terry's Nails

The term *Terry's nails* refers to the fingernail in which the margin of the lunula has migrated out to produce a situation in which the proximal three-quarters or so of the nail is white while the rest is a normal pink band. Many patients with alcoholic cirrhosis have such fingernails, but not all do. Many normal people have such fingernails too, so that this cannot be taken as an important physical sign.

A DECISION WHEEL FOR JAUNDICE

Narrowing the list of causes in any case of jaundice requires the use of relatively few clinical features. It relies far more heavily on laboratory investigations. The most useful clinical features of the complaint are the associated symptoms. Their use is diagrammed in Figure 6-1.

7

BLOOD IN THE STOOL

SPECIFIC FEATURES OF BLOOD IN THE STOOL

Character of Blood in the Stool

Color of Stool

When a patient says he sees blood in the stool he is rarely wrong. The only thing that he can confuse with fresh blood (hematochezia) is a red dietary pigment that might escape digestion. The pigment in beets, if eaten in large quantities, can produce a dark red stool; this is more common in children than in adults. I suppose that other red dietary pigments could cause confusion too. If you are in doubt you can ask if the blood diffuses into the water of the toilet bowl. Fresh blood diffuses rather rapidly and turns the water a familiar light yellowish pink-red color, while beet pigment goes into solution without a change in color.

Many people know that black stools (melena) can mean blood in the stool, so when a patient says he sees blood you should ask if he means black blood, red blood, or something in between ("dark blood"). Blood turns black in the gut lumen because reduced hemoglobin is dark and because bacteria alter the porphyrin pigments. Most of this conversion occurs in the right colon where the colonic bacteria are most active. Thus if blood in the stool looks entirely fresh, its source is the distal one-third of the colon; if it is completely black, its source is likely to be above the cecum; if it is mixed black and red, the source is somewhere in between. This rule holds for low to moderate rates of bleeding. Large-volume bleeding above the cecum creates a loose watery stool because of the osmotic effect of the blood constituents. The flushing of the colon does not give the bacteria time to convert the hemoglobin completely from red to black. Still, the blood rarely looks entirely fresh even in large-volume bleeding from above the cecum.

Black stools can also result from the ingestion of iron, bismuth (usually in Pepto-Bismol), and the excessive intake of spinach and other greens that are cooked and eaten in large quantities by vegetarians and enthusiasts for "ethnic" diets. You must ask about such medicines and foods when you see a patient who complains of black stools.

Stool Volume and Consistency

When a patient says he sees blood in the stools (red, dark red, or black) be sure to ask him about the stool consistency. The osmotic effect of the plasma constituents that escape into the lumen increase the luminal water content and so increase the volume of the luminal contents. The effect depends upon the amount of mucosa exposed to the osmotic effect of the blood and upon the duration of exposure. Thus bleeding into the stomach, small intestine, or right colon regularly increases stool volume and fluidity. Bleeding into the left colon affects volume and fluidity less, depending on how far up in the colon the source is located. Bleeding from the rectum and anal canal has no effect on stool consistency. Remember that the fecal mass is normally well formed by the time it reaches the sigmoid colon. If a grossly bloody stool is also soft and bulky, the bleeding source is likely to be above the sigmoid colon.

Fresh Blood in the Stool: The Relationship of the Blood to the Stool

The fecal mass forms and firms up slowly as it moves along the colon. A bleeding site at a level of the colon where the fecal mass is formed but soft produces a stool in which the blood is mixed into the stool to some degree; blood that comes from a level where the feces is already firm appears mainly to coat the stool surface. You must ask if the blood appears to be mixed into the stool or mainly coats the stool surface.

You must also ask about the temporal relationship of blood and stool. Most patients who complain of blood in the stool are bleeding from a source in the anal canal like hemorrhoids or an anal fissure. With these sources the bleeding occurs when the fragile mucosa in the anal canal is damaged by the passage of a stool, so that the blood mainly comes after the stool has passed. The blood may appear only on the toilet paper or it may be heard or felt to drip into the water in the toilet after the stool has passed. If the blood comes before the stool or if it comes without stool, the source is likely to be above the anal canal.

Chronology of Blood in the Stool

Onset

Blood in the stool is so alarming that most patients know the onset to the day and seek help immediately. The symptom is always abrupt in onset. Unfortunately, some patients seem to think that occasional hematochezia is normal, probably because hemorrhoidal bleeding is so common. Thus they may not mention previous episodes. You must ask about previous hematochezia directly if you want to be sure when the bleeding actually began.

Periodicity

If the bleeding has gone on for more than a short time, it has probably exhibited periodicity. This is characteristic of virtually all causes of rectal bleeding. The lack of periodicity, however, strongly suggests a malignant source, in the left colon if the blood is bright, higher in the colon if the blood is dark and mixed with the stool.

Aggravating and Relieving Factors in Blood in the Stool

Patients rarely can tell you anything they do that aggravates rectal bleeding or that relieves it. Anal-canal bleeding is usually worse with constipation and such bleeding often goes away with treatment of constipation, but not always, since severe hemorrhoidal disease with cryptitis and papillitis is not caused by constipation but it often aggravates constipation.

Associated Symptoms in Blood in the Stool

When rectal bleeding is associated with other major gastrointestinal symptoms the other symptoms usually dominate, but occasionally not so you should ask specifically about them.

The bright or dark-red bleeding of colonic origin frequently occurs without associated symptoms, but you should ask about diarrhea, constipation, and cramps. The diarrhea, if present, is always rather low in volume. It may amount to no more than a consistent increase in stool softness and volume. This suggests an origin above the rectum. Mild constipation coupled with dark blood suggests a neoplasm of the right colon; with bright bleeding it suggests diverticulitis or bleeding of anal-canal origin. Cramps in relation to bright red rectal bleeding are suggestive of a partial colonic obstruction and especially suggest cancer.

The various sources of the black fluid stools produced by bleeding of upper gastrointestinal origin usually lie in the esophagus, stomach, or duodenum, for more distal intestinal sources of bleeding are rare. Ask about *upper-abdominal pain, nausea,* and *cramps* in relation to melena. The gastric lesions that bleed can be either inflammatory or neoplastic, both of which usually cause pain, but not always. Remember that one-fifth of duodenal ulcers are painless and I suspect that one-fifth of gastric cancers and gastric ulcers are too. Nausea and cramps signify that the volume of bleeding is relatively great. Some such symptoms may be present but ignored because they are usually mild. The absence of any upper-abdominal pain, nausea, and cramps suggests that the melena is of cecal or right colonic origin.

THE COMMON CAUSES OF BLOOD IN THE STOOL AS THE MAJOR SYMPTOM

This classification is based on two features of rectal bleeding: the *color of the blood* and the *character of the stool.* The rules on which this classification is based are not infallible.

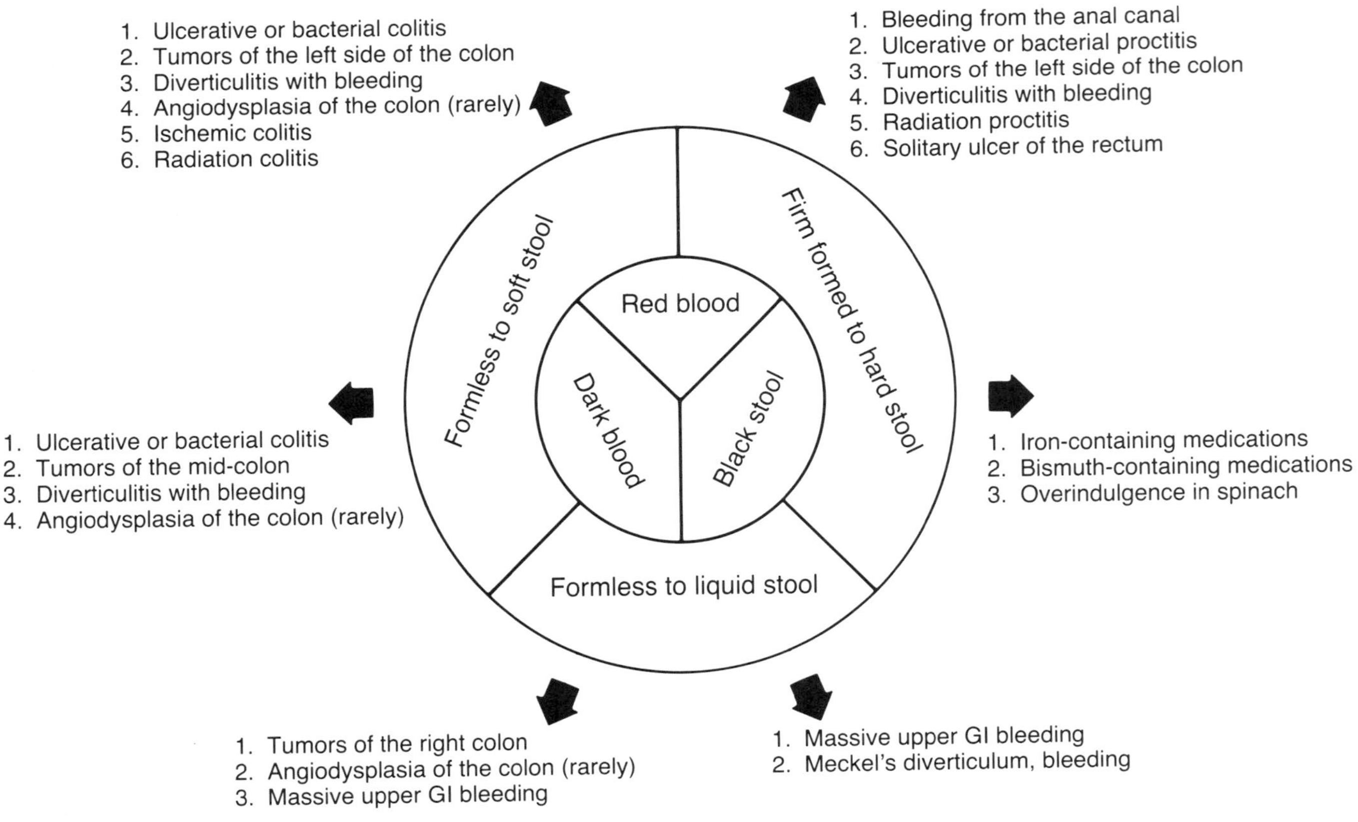

Fig. 7-1. A decision wheel for considering the causes of gross rectal bleeding on the basis of the color of the blood (core) and the consistency of the stool (periphery).

I. Bright red rectal bleeding
  A. The stool is solid and firm
    1. Lesions of the anal canal: hemorrhoids, fissures, carcinomas
    2. Proctitis: idiopathic, traumatic, or bacterial
    3. Adenomas and carcinomas of the left colon
    4. Radiation proctitis
    5. Solitary ulcer of the rectum
  B. The stool is variably soft to formless
    1. Colitis: idiopathic, ulcerative, or bacterial
    2. Adenomas and carcinomas of the mid-colon
    3. Diverticulitis with bleeding
    4. Radiation colitis
    5. The rare case of angiodysplasia of the colon
II. Dark red rectal bleeding
  A. The stool is variably soft to formless
    1. Colitis: idiopathic, ulcerative, or bacterial
    2. Adenomas and carcinomas of the mid-colon
    3. The rare case of angiodysplasia of the colon
    4. Diverticulitis with bleeding
  B. The stool is formless to liquid, but low volume
    1. Adenomas and carcinomas of the right colon
    2. The rare case of angiodysplasia of the colon
III. Black stools which may be interpreted by the patient as bleeding
  A. The stool is solid and firm
    1. The ingestion of iron or bismuth (Pepto-Bismol)
    2. Overindulgence in spinach and other greens
  B. The stool is soft and sticky or liquid and of increased volume
    1. Duodenal ulcer
    2. Gastric cancer or gastric ulcer
    3. Diffuse gastritis
    4. Meckel's diverticulum
    5. Carcinoma of the ampulla

A DECISION WHEEL FOR GROSS RECTAL BLEEDING

Narrowing the list of causes for gross blood in the stool requires relatively few clinical features. It depends far more on endoscopic and radiographic investigations. The important clinical features, the nature of the blood and the nature of the stool, are diagrammed in Figure 7-1.

8

NAUSEA AND VOMITING

WHAT PATIENTS MEAN BY NAUSEA AND VOMITING

Patients do not always know what you mean when you ask about nausea and vomiting. They may use other terms to name the feeling that you would call nausea, calling it a "sick feeling," "queasiness," "indigestion," an "upset stomach," or "urpiness" (in the Middle West). They also may confuse regurgitation with vomiting. Some people think that nausea includes vomiting and so they deny it if vomiting is absent. Other people think that vomiting does not necessarily include nausea and so they describe regurgitation as vomiting.

You have to be clear about what the patient means. I use "queasiness," "a sick feeling," or "sick to the stomach" in asking about nausea. In distinguishing vomiting from regurgitation, I ask if the act of bringing up food or fluid is preceded or accompanied by queasiness or a sick feeling.

THE ORIGIN OF THE SYMPTOM

Nausea usually arises from one of three sources: the abdomen, the brain, and the vestibular apparatus. In abdominal disease the symptom is particularly associated with rapid enlargement of an encapsulated organ or distension of a hollow viscus. This suggests that the responsible nerve endings are mechanoreceptive. The sensation is not apparently produced from esophageal distension, and little or no nausea arises from colonic distension. Thus nausea of abdominal origin usually accompanies sudden distension of the stomach, biliary tract, or intestine and rapid enlargement of the liver or pancreas. Gastric retention occurs in many gastric lesions besides outlet obstruction, like gastritis and gastric motor disturbances, and intestinal dilatation occurs in gastroenteritis and ileus, besides obstruction.

Nausea can also be of central origin, arising from direct excitation of medullary receptors by systemic toxins. This is probably the explanation for the nausea that frequently accompanies many systemic infections and for the nausea of brain tumors and other causes of elevated intracranial pressure. The sensation can also be elicited by vestibular stimulation. When one cause of nausea is mild or subliminal, other nausea-producing stimuli induce more severe nausea. The various inputs to the vomiting center are additive. A patient with gastric outlet obstruction, for example, may feel very nauseated with mild vestibular stimulation like turning the head, which produces no nausea in the normal state.

Vomiting is a complex process, the elements of which are coordinated by the medullary vomiting center. The act involves somatic movements, suspension of respiration, and specific patterns of gastrointestinal contractions. Vomiting is involuntary, triggered when nausea achieves a certain intensity. Whether vomiting accompanies nausea is of little significance. Some people vomit easily and others only with great difficulty.

Regurgitation is different from vomiting in that it is not preceded or accompanied by nausea. It seems to occur whenever the barriers that should prevent it, the esophageal sphincters, do not hold against elevated pressures in the fluid-filled stomach or esophagus.

SPECIFIC FEATURES OF NAUSEA AND VOMITING

The Character of What Comes Up

Patients who bring up anything usually know what it looks, tastes and smells like, but they often fail to volunteer its character to you, so you must ask about it. The character is useful to identify its source.

If the source is the esophagus, solid material predominates. It is food, not very foul-smelling and not very foul-tasting. It may be described as "stringy" because it contains saliva, and the fluid portion is generally colorless.

If the source is the stomach there is usually more fluid than solid material, and the solids, if present at all, look like partly digested food. The fluid is bitter or sour and nasty-smelling. It may or may not be yellow from bile. The taste has been described to me as the feeling that the vomitus "sets my teeth on edge." The absence of bile has some significance. Bile normally flows into the stomach to some degree and is always carried there by intestinal contractions in vomiting. The consistent absence or paucity of bile in bitter vomited or regurgitated material suggests obstruction at the gastric outlet.

If the source of the vomitus is the distal small intestine with a high-grade obstruction, the vomited material sometimes resembles liquid feces. This occurs when colonic bacteria accumulate above the obstructing lesion and flourish in a nutrient medium. Ileal obstruction does not always produce feculent vomiting. It depends on the chronicity of the obstruction. The presence of feculent vomiting is a reliable sign of ileal obstruction. It is rarely a sign of obstruction at any other level of the gut.

Chronology of Nausea and Vomiting

The *onset* and *progress* of nausea and vomiting reflect the onset and progress of the cause. In acute complete bowel obstruction, for example, nausea begins suddenly and progresses rapidly to vomiting. The onset is more insidious in brain tumors and the progress to vomiting is gradual.

When nausea and vomiting occur with no associated symptoms, knowledge of the *circumstances of onset* is not generally useful except in the nausea and vomiting of emotional origin, where you may be able to find that anxiety developed about the time the symptoms began.

The *constancy* of the symptom does not necessarily vary with the nature of the lesion. The most important question in relation to constancy is whether vomiting relieves the nausea. With obstructions in the gut, especially partial obstruction at the gastric outlet, vomiting characteristically relieves the nausea for up to several hours. The failure of vomiting to reduce nausea very much or for very long suggests some cause other than the distension of a hollow viscus that is emptied in vomiting. Such causes include such things as intoxications, brain tumors, or hepatitis.

Aggravating Factors in Nausea and Vomiting

Sometimes you will hear that the nausea occurs mainly or only after eating. This is very characteristic of nausea due to a partial obstruction near the gastric outlet. If the nausea and vomiting occur and persist for hours after a meal it usually represents a gastric outlet obstruction, while their immediate occurrence is more suggestive of gastritis or a gastric ulcer. If you hear a patient say that his nausea comes on mainly after eating, question him about what foods seem to be the worst offenders. Fats, because of their physiologic effect of slowing gastric emptying, can be particularly potent causes of nausea in partial gastric outlet obstruction when other foods are tolerated. In the emptying of a low-fat meal gastric contractions may overcome the partial obstruction, so that the gastric distension does not produce much nausea. A fatty meal, on the other hand, inhibits emptying contractions of the stomach when it reaches the duodenum, and this further distends the stomach to produce nausea. Very fibrous foods occasionally seem to precipitate nausea and vomiting. This is not common, but it can occur if the fiber intake is really excessive. This can precipitate nausea and vomiting in an otherwise asymptomatic case of low-grade gastric outlet obstruction or gastric hypomotility, and in low-grade intestinal obstruction. I have seen this happen in emotionally disturbed or mentally defective patients with pica, in which they consume things like newspaper, cloth, or hair, and in people who overindulge in very fibrous foods like oranges, mushrooms, or water-chestnuts.

Even when nausea is constant in abdominal disease, eating makes the nausea worse. When you hear a clear denial of aggravation of nausea by eating, think especially of nausea due to systemic toxins or intracranial lesions.

When abdominal compression increases the nausea, this strongly suggests intra-abdominal causes. The aggravation of nausea by motion is common to all causes because vestibular stimulation further excites the already-aroused medullary vomiting center. Patients often say that the thought of eating worsens nausea. This, too, occurs in both intra-abdominal and intracranial disease.

Relieving Factors in Nausea and Vomiting

The avoidance of eating or drinking often reduces nausea arising from the hollow viscera. The avoidance of motion reduces nausea of all causes.

Many patients seek relief of nausea by taking antacids. The benefits may represent only a placebo effect, but if the benefit seems to be definite it should make you think of a source related to inflammatory disease of the stomach or duodenum. Also, patients often take one of the many antiemetic drugs. The fact that they help is not useful information in looking for causes.

Associated Symptoms in Nausea and Vomiting

When nausea and vomiting are very prominent, patients often neglect to mention associated symptoms, especially if they are mild, so you must ask specifically about them. Think of four categories of symptoms to ask about or you may forget some: abdominal symptoms, systemic symptoms, cerebral symptoms, and emotional symptoms.

Abdominal Symptoms

Abdominal pain concurrent with nausea points to the abdomen as the source of nausea. Pay particular attention to epigastric pain. Pain can be very mild in gastric and duodenal inflammatory disease so that nausea can be the principal or sole symptom. Crampy pain suggests intestinal obstruction. It is rarely so mild as not to be made evident to you, but it can be.

The changes in diet that nauseated patients make, and the antacids that they take, may produce mild changes in bowel habit. Thus if a nauseated patient acknowledges that he has diarrhea or constipation your interpretation must be cautious. It depends upon the degree and timing of the abnormal bowel habit. Is the diarrhea or constipation a major or a minor problem? Did it begin before the nausea or after? How has your patient tried to treat his nausea? If you judge that the bowel symptoms are not explained by diet and medicines, you are justified in looking for intestinal or colonic causes for nausea, mainly partial intestinal obstructions.

Systemic Symptoms

At the onset of many systemic illnesses, especially viral infections like hepatitis and hematologic or neoplastic disorders like lymphomas, mild nausea is often the chief symptom or the only one. The other symptoms often develop more slowly and later. Symptoms like fever, chills, lassitude, mild headaches, weight loss, and anorexia may be attributed by the patient to the nausea and vomiting, and so he may not tell you about them. You must ask. In evaluating them, you will have special trouble with three: mild headaches, weight loss, and anorexia.

Since a headache alerts you to the thought of raised intracranial pressure,

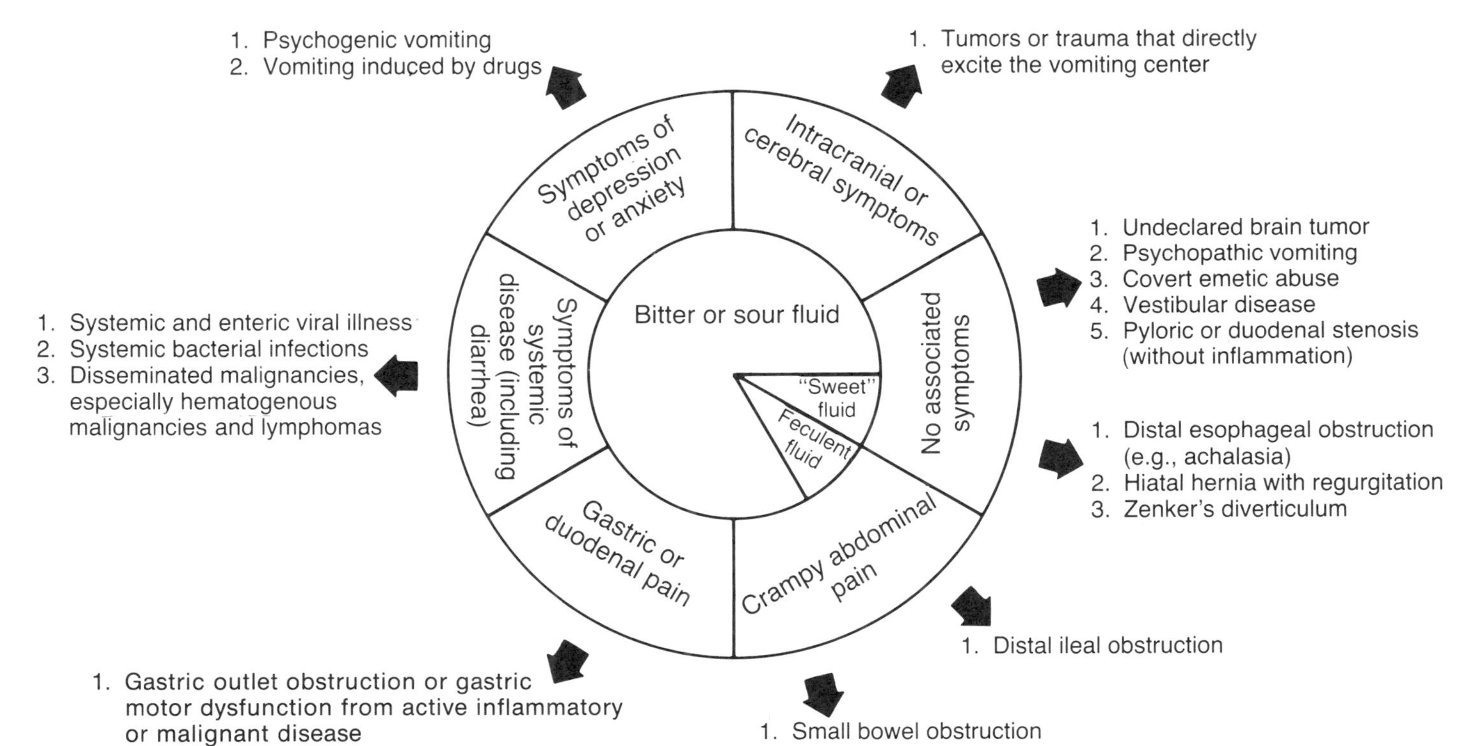

Fig. 8-1. A decision wheel for considering the causes of chronic nausea and vomiting on the basis of the character of the vomitus (core) and the associated symptoms (periphery).

you have to decide if a headache, when present, means that. If a headache, however mild, is the only associated symptom, you should be more concerned about intracranial disease than when other systemic symptoms are also present. When the patient complains of headache you must inquire about other signs of raised intracranial pressure, like somnolence, forgetfulness, clumsiness, visual changes, and hearing loss. The timing of the onset of the headache in relation to that of the nausea is not helpful.

The degree of weight loss and anorexia mean rather little in interpreting nausea. Some anorexia is invariably present with nausea, and weight loss is simply a matter of the duration of the nausea and the degree to which eating is depressed. The timing is more important. If anorexia and weight loss began well before the nausea their significance is much greater, and this should lead you to suspect especially an occult malignancy. When patients complain of severe and prolonged nausea and vomiting with no weight loss, you should suspect anxiety as the cause rather than intra-abdominal disease.

Cerebral Symptoms

A severe headache is a common, but not invariable accompaniment of intracranial causes of nausea. Ask as well about more subtle signs like difficulty with memory, clumsiness, blurred vision, dizziness, and drowsiness. Find out if they began before or after the nausea. Nausea sometimes long precedes other manifestations of brain tumors. The readiness of brain tumors to produce nausea is probably related in part to their proximity to the vomiting center in the brainstem.

Emotional Symptoms

Patients who are depressed or anxious often have anorexia and, not rarely, nausea and vomiting. Some such people successfully conceal other typical symptoms of emotional illness, like sleeplessness, but it is hard to conceal vomiting. Thus nausea is a common presenting complaint in depression and anxiety. Be sure to consult friends or family members about evidence for depression and anxiety when your patient has unexplained chronic nausea as a sole symptom. They may tell you things that the patient himself won't. Patients with anorexia nervosa and bulimia sometimes are brought to you by relatives, with nausea and vomiting as the major complaint. The patients themselves may try to conceal these symptoms or minimize them to you.

A DECISION WHEEL FOR NAUSEA AND VOMITING

Narrowing the list of causes for chronic nausea and vomiting with the use of laboratory examinations can be very difficult. Clinical features can be very helpful. Their use is diagrammed in Figure 8-1.

9

GAS AND BLOATING

INTRODUCTION

Gas and bloating are complaints that commonly bring patients to doctors. Because such complaints often arise from processes that seem trivial to physicians, they may not receive serious consideration in writing, in teaching, or in the clinic. The complaints are not trivial to the patients, however, and they deserve as careful an analysis as any other. Sometimes they herald the onset of serious disease.

WHAT PATIENTS MEAN BY GAS AND BLOATING, AND HOW TO TALK ABOUT THEM

The two terms, *gas* and *bloating*, are often confused by patients because the problems often occur together. You have to find out at the beginning what the exact symptoms are.

You have a problem with terminology in discussing such matters that are somewhat indelicate. When I want to know about what is usually called "gas," I ask about "belching" or "burping" for eructation, and "passing gas" for flatus. In Britain they call the latter problem "wind," and I have heard it called "blowing." I suppose there are many regional slang terms for these two elements of the complaint, some of which are socially acceptable, and you should not hesitate to use them if you are sure you know what they mean. "Bloating" offers less of a problem, but some patients prefer to talk about "abdominal distension," "swelling" of the abdomen, or "feeling full." Women sometimes say "I look like I am pregnant." Use any convenient and acceptable term that the patient uses in talking about the problem because it makes the conversation go much more easily.

The complaint really has three elements: the passage of gas from the stomach by belching, the passage of gas from the anus, and the feeling of abdominal distension. These may occur together in various combinations, or they may occur separately. You must ask about all three elements, their presence or absence, and relative prominence.

THE ORIGIN OF EXCESS BELCHING, FLATUS, AND BLOATING

There is always some gas in the colon because gas is produced there by bacterial fermentation, in the stomach because swallowed air is trapped in the fundus, and in the small bowel because some gastric gas is carried out of the stomach by gastric contractions. Some of this gas is absorbed by diffusion, but much of it is passed through the anus or belched up.

Excessive belching usually means that air is being swallowed in more than usual quantity. Excessive flatus can reflect either the swallowing of too much air or the inordinate production of gas in the colon. The sensation of bloating or abdominal distension can arise from either cause, or it may reflect the presence of excess fluid in the abdomen rather than excess gas. Thus the complaint of gas or bloating should make you think mainly of three processes: excessive air-swallowing, excessive colonic gas production, and excessive intra-abdominal gas and fluid, depending upon which element of the complaint of gas and bloating dominates. A low-grade intestinal obstruction, as occurs in Crohn's disease, can produce bloating as the main complaint.

Excessive Swallowing of Air

Normal people swallow now and then when they are not eating or drinking because anything secreted into the mouth or throat must be disposed of, either by spitting or swallowing. In such swallowing a little air is swallowed as well; air in small quantities also accompanies the bolus in eating and drinking, the more so in drinking carbonated beverages. Excessive air swallowing occurs for the following reasons: (1) *too frequent swallowing* which is often a nervous habit (air-gulping) but may also be a consequence of excess salivary secretion, reflux esophagitis (in which air-swallowing and belching relieve the heartburn), or a chronic nasopharyngeal discharge; (2) *defective chewing,* which is common in people with poor teeth; and (3 *overindulgence in carbonated beverages.*

Excessive Colonic Gas Production

The amount of gas produced by colonic bacterial fermentation depends mainly upon the amount of substrate the bacteria receive. The normal ileal effluent could contain many candidate substrates and it undoubtedly does so, because some gas production seems to occur with virtually any diet. The colon produces excess gas when it receives more than the usual quantity of such substrates, either because of excess intake of fermentable substances or because of defective intestinal absorption.

As for excess intake of substrates, most patients know what foods and drinks are "gassy," like beans and beer, but a few don't; and what is "gassy" for one man is not for another. I do not understand, for example, why overindulgence in cabbage, onions, or nuts engenders flatus in some people but not in others.

As for intestinal malabsorption of fermentable substances, one can be a little more specific. Any intestinal malabsorption or maldigestion can result in excess flatus, usually with at least some change in bowel habit or stool character. Carbohydrate malabsorption, either because of damaged intestinal epithelial cells or brush border disaccharidase deficiency, allows polysaccharides to reach the colon to be fermented.

Excessive Production of Abdominal Fluid

Excess fluid in the abdomen must be located either in the gut lumen or in the peritoneal space. In either case, the unaccustomed volume can produce both the sensations of bloating and of excess gas. Excess belching and flatus probably occur because the fluid takes up space that gas would otherwise occupy. Of course the diarrheal syndromes in which there is an increased fluid volume in the gut lumen are commonly accompanied by excessive flatus because of carbohydrate malabsorption. But when fluid accumulates in the gut lumen for any reason, other symptoms—nausea and vomiting, diarrhea, and cramping abdominal pain—usually dominate the clinical picture. Gas and bloating are relatively minor associated symptoms.

The accumulation of peritoneal fluid—ascites—has many causes. It can occur in relation to any disease that obstructs portal venous flow, hepatic venous outflow, or flow through the inferior vena cava above the hepatic veins. It also occurs in those malignancies that become disseminated in the peritoneal space and secrete fluid. In all these cases, bloating (with or without "gas") is sometimes the initial complaint.

THE SPECIFIC FEATURES OF GAS AND BLOATING

The Character of Gas and Bloating

The complaint can encompass excessive belching, excessive flatus, or a feeling that the abdominal volume is increased; belching, flatus, and girth all vary to some degree normally. Patients rarely count gaseous expulsions or measure the abdomen so that excess can better be defined in terms of a perceptible change than it can be in absolute terms. The definition of abnormality is thus entirely subjective. Patients sometimes confuse excessively foul flatus or belched gas with an excessive volume of gas. It is more noticeable then.

The Chronology of Gas and Bloating

As in all symptoms, the chronology of gas and bloating accurately reflects the chronology of the cause. When the onset is abrupt think of things that change abruptly like the loss of teeth, the recent occurrence of an anxiety-provoking event, or a change in diet. The nature of the onset of a symptom that represents a change in a normal function can be a little fuzzy, so that often you cannot be certain about acuteness. When the onset is insidious think of things that develop slowly. The onset of abdominal distension in malignant ascites is insidious, as is that of portal venous hypertension, but the distension in hepatic venous occlusion is usually more rapid in onset.

Ask about the circumstances of onset. What life events surrounded the onset? Dental work, a change in diet, a move to a new location? In such seemingly trivial matters you may find a simple explanation. You have to be imaginative. I have seen "gas" as the presenting complaint in patients who moved from one location to another where they developed allergic rhinitis with a continuous nasopharyngeal discharge that made for constant swallowing.

Ask about the progress of the complaint. Most causes are fixed and so the complaint tends to be constant rather than periodic. Periodicity most strongly suggests a variability of dietary intake. Unequivocal progression should suggest a progressing problem, like malignant peritoneal effusion or a developing malabsorption syndrome.

Aggravating Factors in Gas and Bloating

Gas and bloating are always more noticed with somatic activity than with inactivity, so knowing that activity is an aggravating factor is not helpful, though most patients mention it. Similarly, eating worsens the symptoms in virtually all causes. Specific foods are worth asking about, but when patients notice specific food intolerances they usually recognize for themselves what to do about it and do not seek your help. Sometimes they don't, though. Patients trying to gain or lose weight may take to eating very strange things in large quantities and they may not relate the onset of gas and bloating to the dietary change. The foods that commonly aggravate gas and bloating, so far as I can determine from talking to patients, are beans, beer, cabbage, lettuce, onions, some green leafy vegetables, nuts, and milk-products in the lactase-deficient. Rapid eating makes for more gas and bloating than leisurely eating, apparently because, for reasons I do not understand, one seems to swallow more air in eating fast. The factor is commonly mentioned in medical texts but it is marginally valid as a sole explanation for gas and bloating.

Relieving Factors in Gas and Bloating

Except for the avoidance of recognized aggravating circumstances, there are none. If any antacid actually relieves the symptoms I would attribute that to a placebo effect, not a physiologic one.

Associated Symptoms in Gas and Bloating

Belching can be associated with delayed gastric emptying so you should find out about gastric symptoms—nausea, postprandial fullness, and epigastric pain. If these symptoms accompany the belching the patient usually mentions

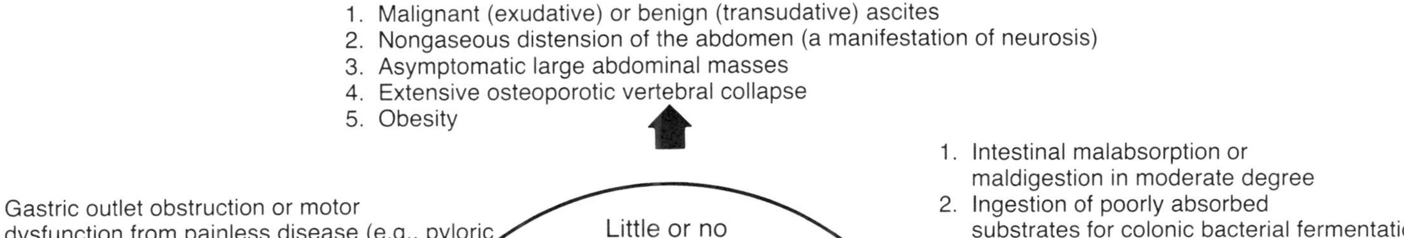
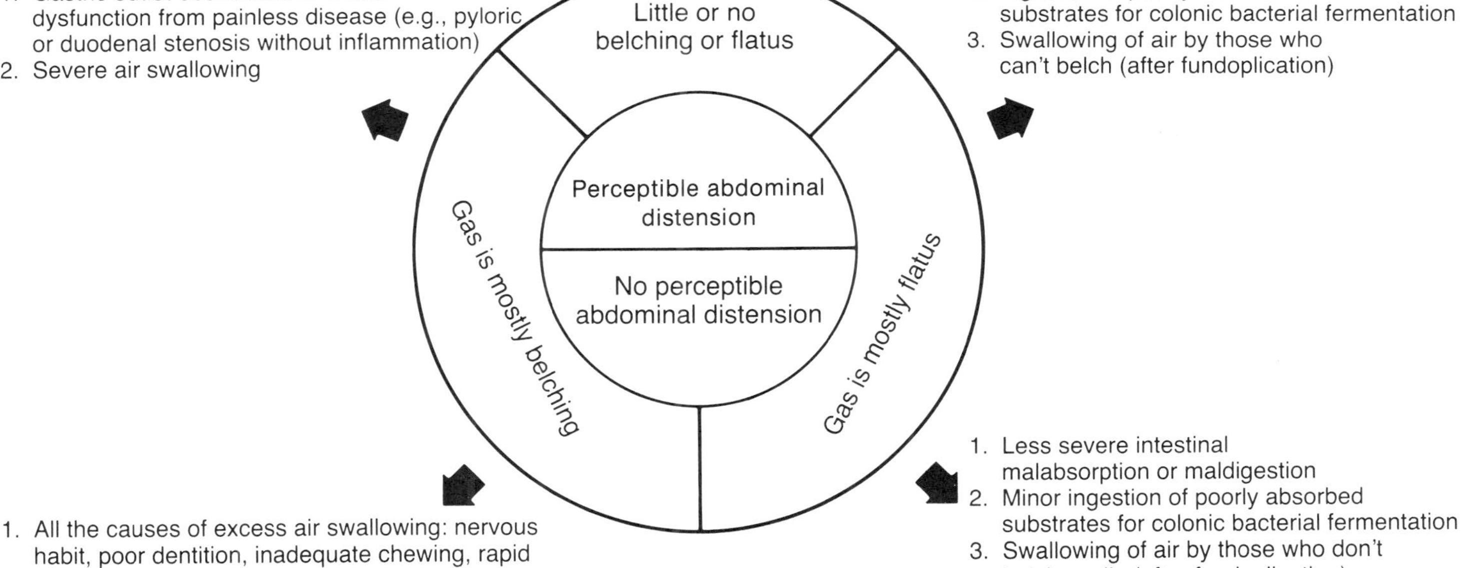

Fig. 9-1. A decision wheel for considering the causes of gas and bloating on the basis of the degree of abdominal distension (core) and what the patient means by "gas" (periphery).

them, and they usually appear as the principal symptom, but you must ask about them if they are not volunteered.

Excessive flatus can be associated with maldigestion and malabsorption, so you should find out about weight loss and increased stool frequency, character, and volume. The change in flatus can precede and dominate the clinical picture in mild maldigestion and malabsorption syndromes so you must always ask about defecation in patients with gas and bloating.

Bowel sounds are aggravated when the gut contains excess gas and fluid. Patients can often hear their own bowel sounds in this situation. You should ask about such borborygmi, but do not call them that. Ask if the patient has noticed that his stomach growls more than usual. This is much more prominent in partial obstruction than it is in air-swallowing.

A DECISION WHEEL FOR GAS AND BLOATING AS A MAJOR COMPLAINT

Narrowing the list of causes for gas and bloating can be quite effectively accomplished by considering some simple clinical features. Their use is diagrammed in Figure 9-1.

10

THE PHYSICAL EXAMINATION IN DIAGNOSTIC GASTROENTEROLOGY

INTRODUCTION

Many textbooks of physical diagnosis describe the techniques and findings of physical examination in diagnostic gastroenterology. My intent in this chapter is to review such usual information, to add or emphasize points that are sometimes neglected, and to relate findings to anatomy and physiology more than to nosologic entities. I have avoided using eponyms for physical signs: They are not descriptive, their use clouds physiologic thinking, and they tend to confuse the novice.

THE ABDOMINAL EXAMINATION

How to Begin the Abdominal Examination

In examining the abdomen you must apply the usual methods of physical examination in a particular order: inspection, auscultation, palpation, and percussion. Auscultation precedes palpation because palpation may stimulate intestinal contractions, the sounds of which obscure vascular sounds.

When the body is fully supine the abdominal wall is flattened. This is the best *position of the abdomen* for inspection and auscultation, and so the patient should first be put in this position. Palpation is facilitated by a relaxed abdomen so that, after auscultation, you should put the patient with his trunk in a slightly flexed position to reduce the tension of the abdominal wall. You can accomplish this either or both by raising the chest and flexing the hips and knees. You should raise the head of the bed or examining table when this is possible, or put pillows under the patient's head and shoulders. You can produce flexion of the hips and knees by putting pillows under the knees.

A surface map of the abdomen is sometimes used to describe the location of abnormalities. There are two systems of mapping. In the simpler system you divide the abdomen into quadrants by drawing two imaginary lines through the umbilicus, one in the craniocaudad axis and the other transverse. The four regions created are called the right and left upper quadrants and the right and left lower quadrants (Fig. 10-1A). In the more complex and less-used system extensions of the nipple lines across the abdomen are transected by two transverse lines, one connecting the two costal margins at their most caudad points and the other connecting the two superior iliac crests. This produces nine regions, called the right and left hypochondria, the epigastrium, the right and left flanks, the periumbilical region, the right and left inguinal regions, and the suprapubic region (Fig. 10-1B). In practice I find it more natural to think of organs than of regions delineated by such surface maps. Thus later in the chapter, I commonly refer to regions of organs or to specific organs rather than to quadrants or segments based on surface maps.

Inspection of the Abdomen

How to Look at the Abdomen

Inspection of the abdomen should include inspection with oblique lighting. If the oblique light is stationary, it works well if it is placed over the head of the patient, directed toward his feet. I find it useful to have a movable light source, like a flashlight, to use in a darkened room. You should walk around the patient, pointing the light as necessary. Oblique light is important because enlarged organs can often be seen to cast a shadow if the light is arranged properly. This is especially useful to see a distended gallbladder. This use of oblique light is only temporary, and you should use overhead light for the rest of the inspection.

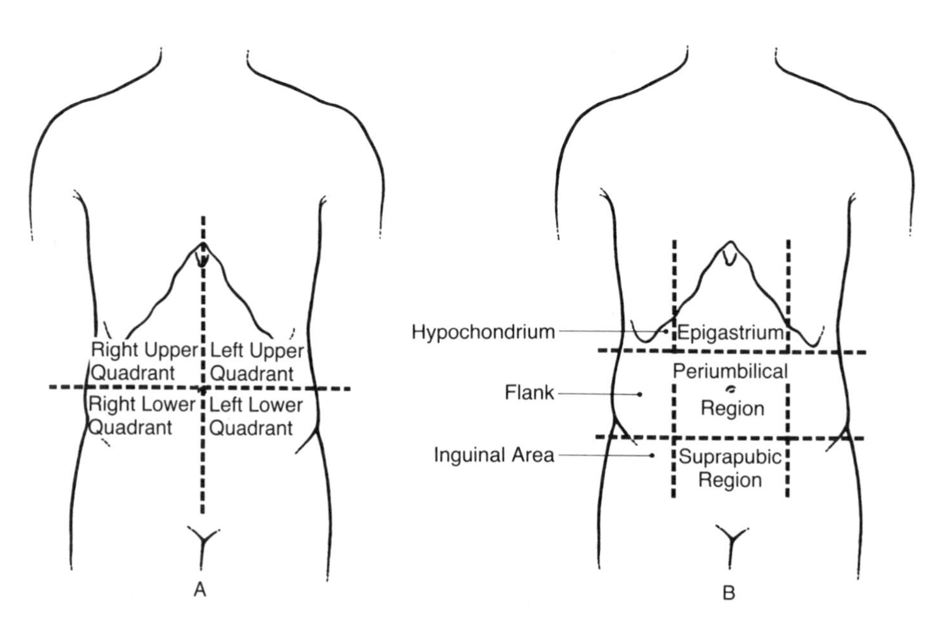

Fig. 10-1. (A & B) The two systems of mapping the surface of the abdomen.

Configuration of the Abdomen

You should first note the configuration of the abdomen (Fig. 10-2). In most people with normal musculature the abdominal wall sinks slightly within the bony margins of the abdominal surface to produce a boatlike ("scaphoid") configuration. In very muscular people you can see the margins of the rectus muscles (the most superficial abdominal wall muscles) with the surface indentations of these muscles produced by the rectus inscriptions, the fibrous bands that traverse these muscles. These inscriptions and the lateral edges of these muscles can be mistaken for the edges of organs in palpation (Fig. 10-3) and so their prominence and location should be assessed at inspection. The medial edges of the two rectus muscles are normally contiguous at the midline, but they may be variably separated, either as a congenital variation or as a result of pregnancy, obesity, or ascites. You should look for such a separation, *diastasis recti,* at inspection, for the displaced medial edges of the muscles can also be mistaken for abnormal intra-abdominal masses. You should ask the patient to raise his head from the pillow. The resultant contraction of the rectus muscles and the rise in intra-abdominal pressure bulges the fascia between the separated recti and reveals a diastasis if it is present.

In those with normal musculature and a normal nutritional state, the abdo-

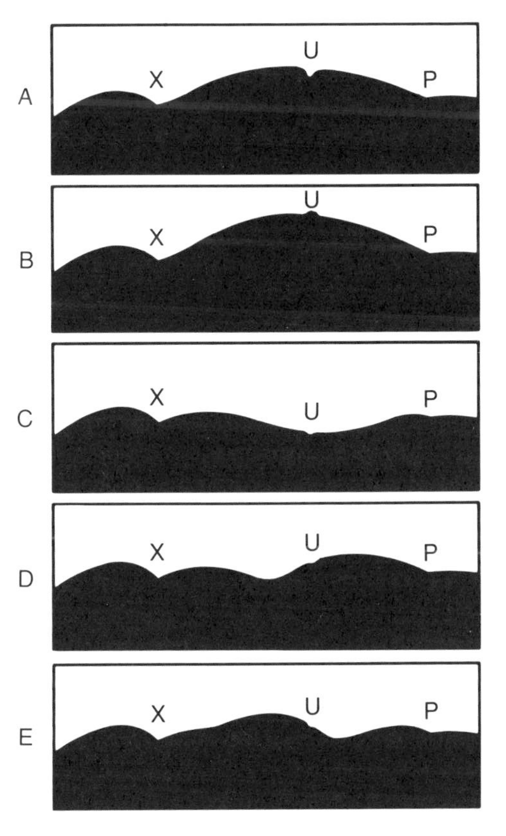

Fig. 10-2. The various configurations of the abdominal silhouette. In all silhouettes, *X* is the xiphoid process, *U* is the umbilicus, and *P* is the pubis. (**A**) The configuration of the abdomen in obesity or gaseous distension: the umbilicus is inverted. (**B**) The configuration in ascites: the umbilicus is everted. (**C**) The scaphoid (boat-shaped) configuration of slender people. (**D**) The configuration in the presence of a lower abdominal mass, a distended bladder for example. (**E**) The configuration in the presence of an upper abdominal mass, an enlarged liver, for example.

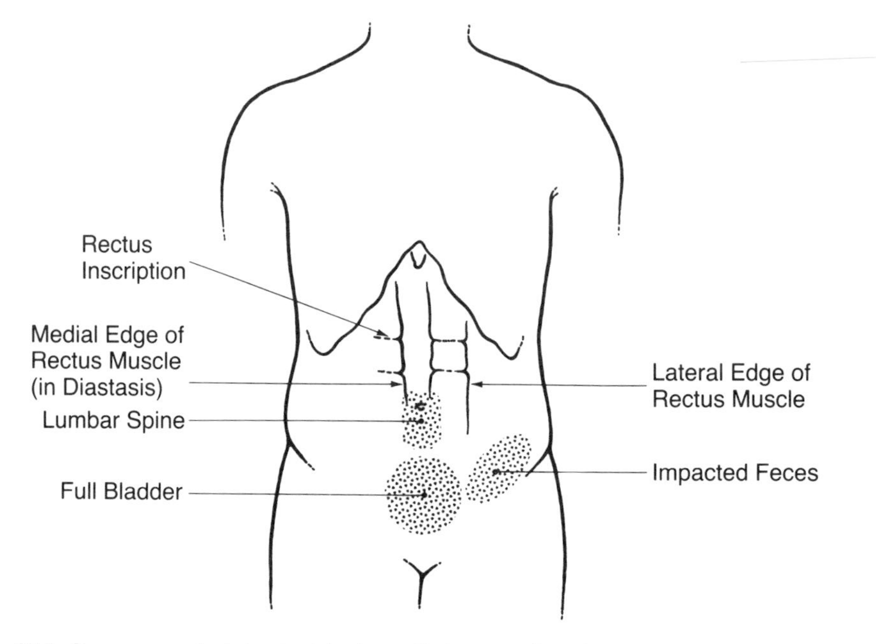

Fig. 10-3. Some normal abdominal features that are easily mistaken for abnormal masses. These include the rectus inscriptions, the lateral edge of the rectus, the medial edge of the rectus in diastasis recti, the lumbar spine, a full urinary bladder, and fecal impaction.

men has a slightly rounded contour. When this rounded contour appears to be greater than normal, the abdomen is said to be bulging or protuberant. This may be due to fat, gas, ascites, intra-abdominal tumors, or a feces-packed colon. You can sometimes distinguish among these by the configuration of the flanks. When generalized abdominal enlargement is due to fat or intra-abdominal masses the bulging at the flanks has a rolled appearance in cross-section, while ascites and gas produce a smoother curvature suggesting the surface of an inflated balloon (Fig. 10-4).

The surface of the abdomen is normally symmetrical right-to-left. Distension may be localized to one region to produce right-to-left asymmetry in the case of an abnormal mass or a distended or enlarged organ. You can assess symmetry by standing either behind the head or at the feet of the patient and comparing the two sides. Retraction of surgical scars and the presence of masses in the abdominal wall also produce asymmetry.

A greatly enlarged or distended organ may be visible on the abdominal surface as a shadow cast by oblique light. The position of the shadow suggests the organ that is enlarged. When you see such shadows in the upper quadrants, you can see them move with respiration if the enlarged organ lies adjacent to the diaphragm and is not fixed to retroperitoneal structures. The edge of an enlarged liver is often visible and shows respiratory motion. An enlarged spleen also moves with breathing, but it is harder to see. A very distended stomach is sometimes visible. It moves less with respiration because it is deformed rather

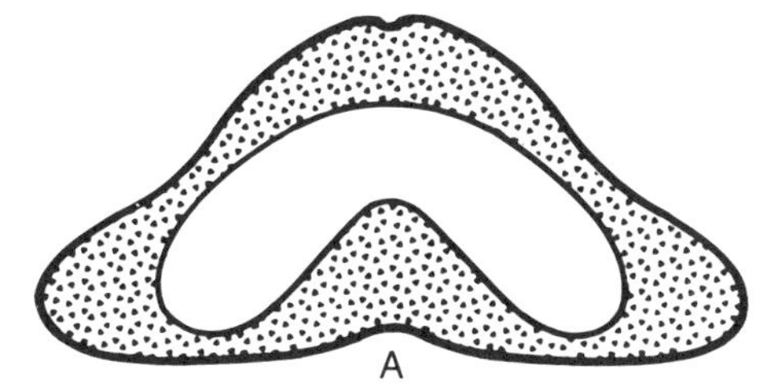

Fig. 10-4. The configuration of the flanks in obesity (**A**) contrasted with that in distension from ascites or gas (**B**).

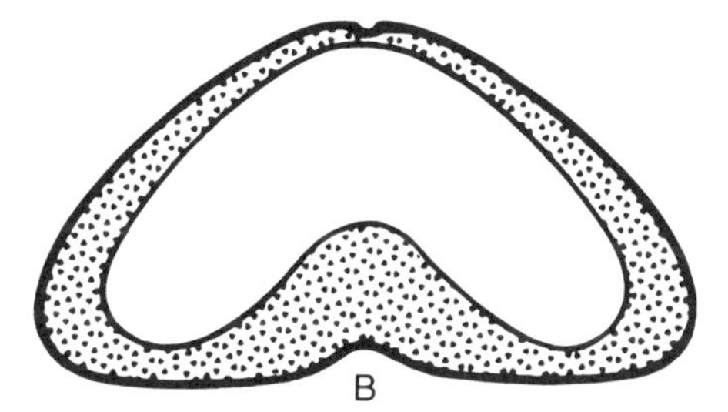

than displaced by diaphragmatic motion. A gallbladder that is enlarged because of obstruction at its outlet may be easier to see than it is to feel, appearing as a small globular enlargement in the right upper quadrant that moves with respiration. Shadows cast by localized organ distensions in the lower abdomen do not move with respiration. The position of such a shadow or visible mass suggests the organ that is involved. A distended urinary bladder appears as a globular mass in the midline that can extend to the umbilicus in extreme cases. An enlarged uterus may also be visible as a midline mass. Visible masses in the lower quadrants are rare. They usually represent lesions related to the colon or ileum. In very slender people an enlarged kidney may be visible lateral to the umbilicus. It usually moves little with respiration.

The Umbilicus

The normal umbilicus is symmetrically indented into the abdominal wall, though it may be nearly flat in very slender people. An everted umbilicus is always abnormal. It is the result of herniation at the fascial opening of the umbilicus. Eversion is very common in ascites, particularly in extreme degrees of ascites, but it may also represent only herniation of bowel or fat into a widened umbilical ring. If you see an everted umbilicus you should ask how long it has been present. That may suggest the nature of the cause. Rarely, the umbilicus exudes fluid. Umbilical drainage of ascitic fluid can occur in massive ascites, and drainage of feculent material occurs when enteric fistulas have formed to the umbilicus; fistulas can occur in inflammatory and malignant lesions. You will occasionally see umbilical nodules. They are usually lipomas, but they can represent metastasis or extension of intra-abdominal malignancy. Umbilical stones are concentrations of dirt and desquamated epidermis that form in those of neglected toilet.

The Abdominal Skin

Examine the skin color over the abdomen with strong light. The lower abdomen is rarely exposed to the sun, so that disorders characterized by generalized hyperpigmentation may be quite evident there. Also, mild degrees of jaundice that are easily concealed by a suntan may be most apparent in the lower abdomen. Look at the color of the skin in the flanks in those who give a history of abdominal pain. In any condition that has produced massive retroperitoneal bleeding (classically in hemorrhagic pancreatitis) the blood dissects around the flanks between the fascial layers below the subcutaneous fat, to reach the subepidermal tissue on the anterior abdomen, either in the flanks or about the umbilicus. When this is recent the skin in these areas is black-and-blue; later, the color changes to brown or yellow, and this may persist for many days. In fact, this is not seen in all cases of retroperitoneal hemorrhage. It signifies massive retroperitoneal bleeding.

Abdominal striae, commonly called "stretch-marks," are common on the abdomen. They represent the rupture of subepidermal connective tissue as a result of abdominal distension, either recent or remote. When they first form, striae are reddish or pink; if the state of distension stabilizes or the cause regresses, the color fades to white over about 6 months, except when striae form as a result of the taking of large doses of corticosteroids. In that case they remain pink until the dosage is reduced. The location of the striae sometimes suggests the locus of the distending lesion. Striae due to pregnancy are prominent in the lower abdomen while those due to generalized abdominal enlargement or massive corticosteroid usage are more widespread, but they are often most prominent in the flanks.

You should examine abdominal scars carefully. Scars, like striae, are reddish-pink for about 6 months after they form and then usually fade to white. The location and size of a scar suggest the nature of the operation that was done. For example the characteristic scar of a McBurney's incision indicates that the surgeon who made it strongly suspected and found uncomplicated appendicitis and that he did very little further exploration of the abdomen. It is useful to talk over each surgical scar with the patient. This may reveal operations or findings that the patient neglected to mention to you in your review of his operations. The locations of incisions commonly used for abdominal operations are shown in Fig. 10-5. Be sure to look at scars left by drains. They may also suggest what was done (T-tube drainage of the common bile duct, for example), or reveal that an operation was complicated by infection. Ask the patient about these drains, how long they were present, and what kind of fluid drained from them.

Abdominal abrasions are often a manifestation of scratching in generalized pruritus when they are not seen elsewhere. The abdomen does not itch more than other regions, but it is easier to reach. You will sometimes see abdominal

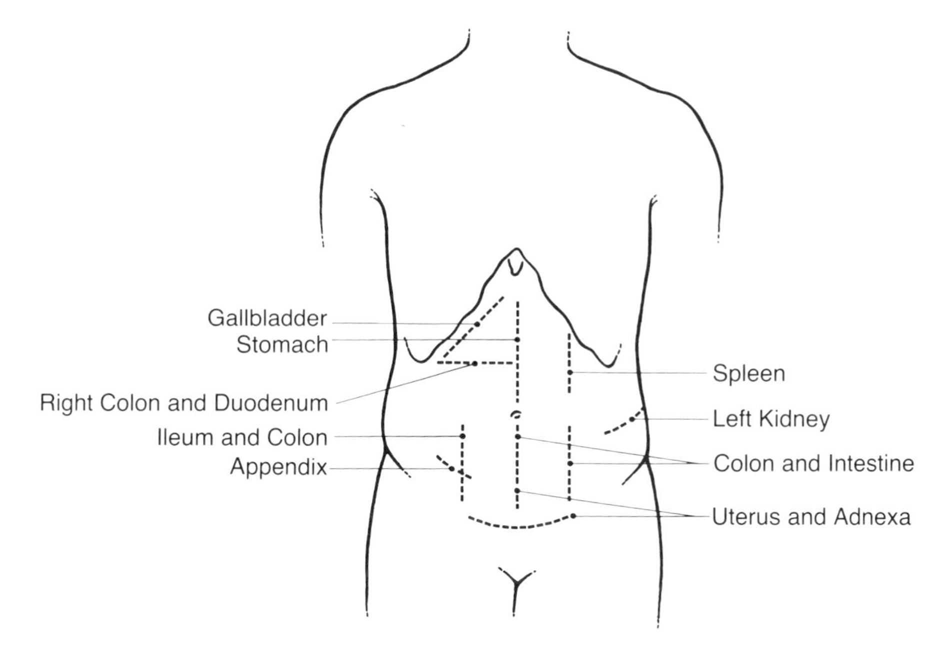

Fig. 10-5. Some common surgical scars and what they can suggest about the organ that was attacked. Vertical (cephalocaudad) incisions are generally made to give broad exposure. The choice between midline and paramedian vertical incisions rests more on custom than on practical considerations of access.

abrasions in patients with generalized abdominal distension of rapid onset, since rapid stretching of the skin can make it itch.

The Veins of the Anterior Abdominal Wall

The veins of the abdominal wall are usually not visible, but normal veins may be conspicuous in thin or old people. Veins may become visible when the skin is stretched by generalized abdominal distension. When the veins are abnormally distended you can usually see them easily. The fact that veins can be seen is not useful, but the direction of blood flow in visible veins can be useful information because these veins connect to the portal system through the umbilical vein. To demonstrate the direction of flow, first occlude a visible vein with your two index fingers side-by-side and then slide them apart to empty a short length of the vein. Then lift one finger before the other and repeat the maneuver, lifting the other finger first. This way you can discover if the vein fills from one direction or the other. This works because these veins lack valves. Blood in these veins normally flows *away* from the umbilicus, cephalad above the umbilicus and caudad below it (Fig. 10-6). Obstruction of the inferior vena cava below the hepatic veins produces reversal of flow (toward the umbilicus) in the *lower* abdomen; superior vena caval obstruction produces flow reversal (toward the umbilicus) in the *upper* abdomen. Reversed flow is much faster than antegrade

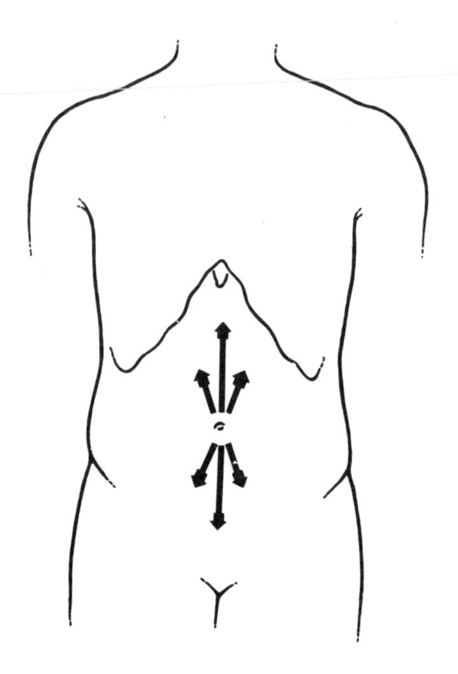

Fig. 10-6. The normal direction of flow in the superficial abdominal veins. Flow is normally away from the umbilicus.

flow. Portal venous obstruction does not affect the direction of flow, but the exaggerated venous flow through the umbilical vein in portal obstruction may produce greater prominence of those veins adjacent to the umbilicus than of those remote from it.

Visible Peristalsis

You may occasionally see regularly recurring rippling movements across the abdominal wall that are instantly recognizable as visible peristalsis. This appearance may be normal in people who are emaciated or very thin, but it is abnormal in patients who have normal adiposity and it is an important sign in those who have a pattern of abdominal pain that is suggestive of an intestinal obstruction. Visible peristalsis usually originates in the small intestine, since that organ underlies most of the anterior abdominal wall, but the waves may also be of gastric or colonic origin. The organ of origin can be inferred from the location of the visible peristalsis and from the frequency; rhythmic gastric peristalsis has a maximal period of 20 seconds, while rhythmic intestinal peristalsis has a maximal period of 5 to 8 seconds. Gastric peristalsis is commonly seen in neonates with congenital hypertrophic pyloric stenosis, probably because neonates have relatively big stomachs and little fat, but it is rarely visible in adults with gastric outlet obstruction. You may see intestinal peristalsis in partial and chronic intestinal obstruction, but less commonly in acute or complete obstruction because of the resultant ileus. Colonic obstruction is usually not manifest as visible peristalsis.

Visible Pulsations

You can often see pulsation of the aorta in the abdomen. The pulsation is more conspicuous in the thin than in the fat, and greater in the old than in the young. It is increased in patients who have a widened pulse pressure (as in thyrotoxicosis, hypertension, or aortic regurgitation), in those with a tortuous aorta, in those with an aortic aneurysm, and in those who have a mass joining the aorta to the anterior abdominal wall. Thus visualization of the aortic pulse is not necessarily abnormal. You must try to judge its force. Judging its force is difficult by inspection alone and requires palpation.

Auscultation of the Abdomen

How to Listen to the Abdomen

Auscultation takes time if it is to be productive. Auscultation in routine examinations is not often rewarding so it may be neglected or done in a cursory fashion. On the other hand it can give a clue to vascular disease or supplement other information that suggests specific disease processes.

You must sit down and place the diaphragm of the stethoscope on the abdomen without holding it in place. You should not press the diaphragm into the abdomen. This maneuver will only slightly amplify sounds and it leads you to listen too briefly. Also, you can produce a bruit by pressing too hard on the aorta. Warm the stethoscope at the tap or in your hand before you start. You should listen at any spot for several minutes. Vascular sounds may be very faint, and you must concentrate for a long time to hear them. Normal intestinal sounds are intermittent and often infrequent. In deciding that bowel sounds are absent you should listen for at least 5 minutes. If the sound of movement of abdominal hair on the diaphragm is a problem, you can minimize this by applying lubricating jelly to the stethoscope diaphragm.

Where to listen is important. Bowel sounds are generalized so they can be assessed adequately by listening in one place, usually just above the umbilicus. Vascular sounds are usually well localized (Fig. 10-7). You should keep the specific locations of vascular sounds in mind and you should listen at all such sites, particularly when the history has suggested to you that vascular sounds may be present.

Arterial Sounds

Arterial sounds in the abdomen, called *bruits,* are sometimes heard in the absence of significant vascular disease, rarely in the young, more often in the elderly. These are variably harsh sounds, easily recognized as arterial because they occur in tempo with the pulse. As elsewhere, such sounds represent turbulence in arterial flow. Turbulence is a consequence of interruption of laminar flow by unusually acute angulations at arterial branch points, by arteriosclerotic plaques, by extreme tortuosity of an artery, or by compression of an artery by

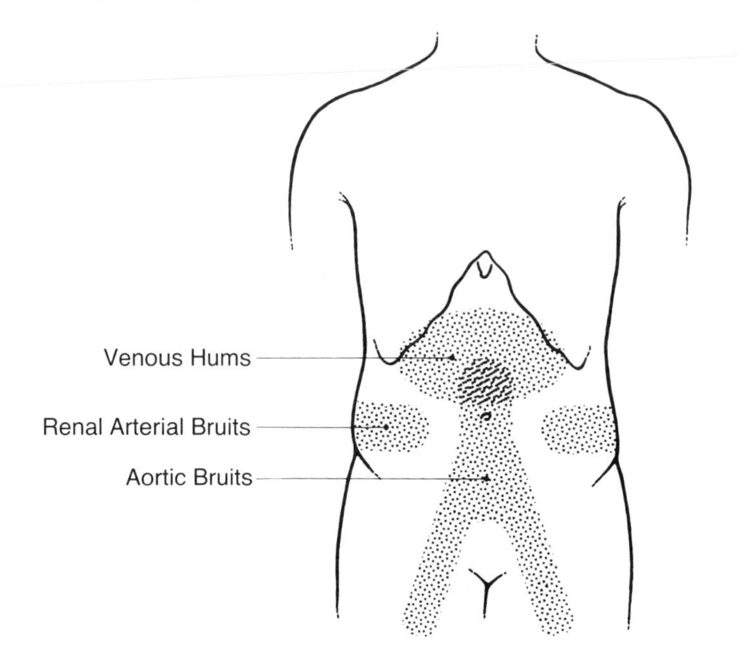

Fig. 10-7. Areas in the abdomen where sounds of vascular origin are most commonly heard.

solid organs or masses. Bruits can also reflect the massive blood flow through very vascular tumors like hepatomas or hemangiomas. Bruits most commonly occur over the aorta, the splenic artery, and the renal arteries. You can also hear bruits over the liver and spleen. Because bruits may occur in the normal abdomen, you need to decide what to consider abnormal.

Bruits over the liver and spleen should always be considered to be abnormal. Over the liver, they signify an unusually vascular tumor like a hepatoma or an angioma. Over the spleen, they may also represent an unusually vascular tumor or hemangioma; splenic bruits can represent transmission of a bruit of splenic arterial origin, in which case the bruit can usually be heard along the course of the splenic artery toward the midline of the abdomen.

Bruits over the aortic area, when they are soft, have no significance; a very loud bruit may represent extensive atherosclerosis, extreme tortuosity of the aorta, or an aortic aneurysm. The transmission of an aortic bruit into the iliac arteries or femoral arteries more strongly suggests significant aortic disease than when such transmission is absent. In the interpretation of a loud and transmitted aortic bruit, the principal consideration is the question of the existence of an aortic aneurysm. The answer to this question is made easier by palpation of the aorta.

Bruits over the renal arteries may occur in the presence or absence of an aortic bruit. These are often best heard in the flanks. Such a bruit is usually an abnormal finding signifying renal arterial stenosis, an important cause of hypertension. But renal arterial stenosis does not very often cause a renal arterial bruit.

Venous Sounds

Sounds arising from venous flow in the abdomen, called *venous hums,* are uncommon. A venous hum in the abdomen is always abnormal. You can distinguish it from an arterial bruit because it is more or less continuous and it is usually softer and lower-pitched than a bruit. A venous hum arises from flow in the portal venous system. It signifies portal-systemic shunting of venous flow when portal flow is obstructed. Such shunts are particularly abundant or accessible in the upper abdomen so venous hums are usually heard there, especially in the area of the liver itself, over the umbilicus, and above the umbilicus where the falciform ligament and umbilical vein lie.

Vascular Sounds Transmitted from the Chest

The murmur of *aortic valvular stenosis* is commonly transmitted along the course of the aorta, and so extremely loud aortic valvular murmurs may be transmitted into the abdomen. You can discover the cardiac source of such a sound by listening to the heart.

Intestinal Sounds

Sounds generated by the contractions of the muscular walls of the gut come from the vibration of the gut wall produced by the movement of a gas–fluid mixture through the gut. Because such a mixture is usually present, the normal gut continuously generates such sounds, called bowel sounds. They persist in fasting because of the presence of gastrointestinal secretions and swallowed air. Most bowel sounds are generated by the small intestine.

Normal bowel sounds vary in quantity. The incidence and loudness of bowel sounds are related to the quantity of swallowed air and the time since the last meal. If loud bowel sounds accompany cramping abdominal pain or abdominal distension, this concurrence suggests partial bowel obstruction.

More significance is attached to the absence of bowel sounds. The absence of bowel sounds for a full 5 minutes strongly suggests the existence of intestinal atony or ileus, which has many causes.

Bowel sounds vary greatly in pitch and quality, being low-pitched or high-pitched gurgles or rumbles. "Tinkling" bowel sounds represent bowel obstruction. If they are present they occur only briefly between long intervals of silence. They constitute a series of faint, high-pitched musical notes with a damped bell-like character, occurring in a brief series of about eight or ten in rather regular sequence—"tink-tink-tink." These are not always heard to interrupt the silence of bowel obstruction, but their presence is certainly consistent with obstruction. The mechanism of origin of these sounds is not known.

Succussion Splash

A large volume of fluid and air may collect in the stomach. You can shake the abdomen and hear the splash at the fluid–gas interface, often without a stethoscope. You can hear this easily in a normal person who has recently eaten or drunk a reasonable volume; it occurs long after meals in cases of gastric outlet obstruction.

Peritoneal Friction Rub

The viscera near the diaphragm move with respiration and rub peritoneal surfaces together. When there is peritonitis in the upper abdomen without much exudate, the rubbing of the inflamed peritoneal surfaces produces a friction rub with respiration. This is a dry, soft, scraping sound exactly like that of a pleural friction rub. It is a rare finding, heard only early in the course of peritonitis. The sound sometimes occurs in splenic infarction, in neoplastic disease that involves the surface of the liver, and in abscess formation in either organ. You can often hear it after needle biopsy of the liver, where it signifies a hemorrhage at the hepatic surface.

Survey Palpation of the Abdomen

The Purpose and Technique of Survey Palpation

Palpation is the most important part of the abdominal examination. In palpation you can discover the size and shape of normally palpable organs, find normally impalpable organs, discover palpable masses that are not normally present, and detect the location and degree of tenderness. You should palpate the abdomen in two stages: survey palpation, described in this section, and specific palpation.

Accuracy in palpation requires the proper position of the patient and the examiner. The patient should be supine with some flexion of the dorsal spine to relax the tension of the anterior abdominal wall. You should raise his head and shoulders a few inches and slightly flex his knees and hips. You can do this easily with modern adjustable beds and examining tables or with pillows.

You should always approach the abdomen from the patient's right side. This may be only convention, but it is universally observed, and when you learn palpation from that approach you cannot conveniently do it from the left side. Careful palpation requires that you be comfortable, relaxed, and patient. I find that it works well if I sit down when I want to feel something very carefully.

Most patients expect abdominal palpation to be uncomfortable and protectively tense the abdominal muscles in anticipation of or in response to the first touch. You can minimize this effect by some simple maneuvers. You should explain that you know that you may produce some discomfort, that you want to minimize this, and that you will be gentle and considerate. You should warm your hands at the tap, since cold hands on the abdomen always elicit protective responses.

Some patients are very ticklish and you will discover this immediately. In this case you should ask the patient to rest his hand on the back of your examining hand and to follow it about the abdomen. This works because of the fact, familiar to all children, that one cannot tickle himself.

Survey palpation is intended to discover the general state of things in the abdomen. You should leave specific features for the later specific palpation of the abdomen. You never want to elicit severe pain or discomfort in survey palpation for fear of setting up protective abdominal responses.

You should use only one hand, your dominant hand, in survey palpation because you control motion of that hand better and because you feel things better with the fingertips of that hand.

Tenderness

One objective of survey palpation is to find areas of tenderness. Usually the history will have suggested regions where tenderness is to be expected, and so you should begin palpation at any other location, reserving the area of tenderness to the last. If you expect no tenderness you should begin by asking if some area is tender or painful and proceed accordingly. If the patient does not know of any tender area, make a very light survey of the four quadrants with your examining hand. You should palpate with the four fingers of the examining hand held contiguously with the fingertips in the same plane, pressing very lightly, just enough to indent the abdominal surface. Then move your hand about, pressing similarly to cover the whole abdomen. Talk to the patient continuously, asking about tenderness and explain what you are doing. Encourage him to relax, to "let go," continuously as you palpate. When you find tenderness, move away from that area, reserving that area until last. In this way you can quickly create a mental map of the abdomen to indicate where tender areas are located.

You should seek *percussion tenderness* in survey palpation when tenderness seems to be extreme. Remember that you want to be very gentle in people with great tenderness. The presence of tenderness in response to gentle percussion has the same significance as the presence of rebound tenderness (peritoneal irritation), and it is a far kinder technique. When you find percussion tenderness do not proceed to look for rebound tenderness.

Resistance to Pressure

Another objective of the survey palpation is to detect areas of resistance to light pressure. The normal abdomen exerts a sensation of resistance to light pressure that is spongy and uniform in all areas except over the liver where the resistance is slightly increased (if the liver lies far enough below the right costal margin). A similar slight increased resistance or hardness anywhere else in the abdomen is abnormal. You should quickly make a mental map of the locations of any areas of resistance to light survey palpation.

Generalized increased resistance to pressure over the whole abdomen suggests several things. It may only represent "guarding," tension of the abdominal muscles in anticipation of discomfort. In that case it should diminish as you get the patient to relax. In ascites the abdomen feels a little like a water-filled balloon. When the bowel is distended by fluid or gas, the belly may feel slightly firmer than the normal spongy abdomen. Great rigidity (usually called a "boardlike abdomen") signifies generalized peritonitis reflecting reflex spasm of the abdominal musculature. Pancreatobiliary secretions are far more irritating to the peritoneum than bacteria are, and so boardlike rigidity suggests a chemical peritonitis, most commonly due to a perforated duodenal or gastric ulcer. Bacterial peritonitis rarely produces a boardlike abdomen until late in its course, and it may be accompanied by only a little increased resistance to compression.

Other Things to Feel in Survey Palpation

In survey palpation you should feel anything else that seems unusual or notable. You should find out if cutaneous eruptions are nodular or sore. You should feel subcutaneous nodules to see if they are soft like lipomas, hard like leiomyomas and malignant tumors, or tender, as in superficial abscesses or hematomas. You should test dilated superficial abdominal veins to discover the direction of filling. You should feel along other scars to discover if they are tender, indicating local infection, contain wire sutures, which feel like wire and may be tender, contain exquisitely tender firm nodules, suggesting neuromas, or contain soft compressible masses, representing local herniations. You should feel the umbilicus for nodules and assess the size of the umbilical ring.

Specific Palpation of the Abdomen

The Purpose and Technique of Specific Palpation

In specific palpation of the abdomen you further explore abnormalities that you found or suspected from the inspection, auscultation, and survey palpation and you explore other matters that are routine parts of the abdominal examination. You can use one hand for both light and deep palpation, but it is better to use both hands in deep palpation. In this case the functions of your two hands differ: You use your dominant hand to feel and your subordinate hand to exert pressure. Put your subordinate hand on the back of your dominant hand to press it into the abdomen. When I press deeply with the hand that I am also using for feeling, that seems to blunt my perception. In some locations you can use your subordinate hand to press a movable organ into a position where your dominant hand can feel it. This is called *ballottement.*

Tenderness

Degree

You must judge the degree of tenderness from what the patient says or how he reacts to elicited discomfort. Tenderness that is moderate or severe always signifies an inflammatory state. Tumors and solid organs enlarged by noninflammatory processes are often not tender at all, or only slightly so. Judgment of the degree of tenderness requires consideration of the character of the patient. Watch the patient's face as you palpate his abdomen. Some patients are stoic and minimize pain, others are sensitive and maximize it, and a few seem to enjoy it. Many normal people are tender to deep palpation over the cecum, sigmoid colon, and aorta. You should tell people who are tender in these areas that this is not necessarily abnormal.

Location

You should map the location of tenderness carefully with as much discrimination as possible. First you should find the margins of the tender area. Then you should go over the area to discover the point of maximal tenderness. You can do this best by rather deep palpation with one finger, pressing at as many points as may be necessary and observing the degree of tenderness. The resulting map can be very useful in establishing the source of the tenderness and its extent. The location of the point of maximal tenderness suggests the organ of origin.

Depth

You should gauge the depth of tenderness. Tenderness can arise from any depth beneath your compressing finger. You can judge the depth from the degree of compression required to elicit discomfort. When only very light pressure is required, this is called *superficial tenderness;* when great pressure is required, this is called *deep tenderness.* Superficial tenderness can arise from the skin, the subcutaneous tissues, the muscle or fascia of the abdominal wall, the anterior parietal peritoneum, or a very tender organ that lies next to the anterior abdominal wall. Deep tenderness signifies a source that is not adjacent to the abdominal wall; it may even be retroperitoneal.

It is very important for you to decide if superficial tenderness has its origin in the abdominal wall or in the intra-abdominal viscera. The way to do this is to ask the patient to raise his head, or both his head and heels, and hold them in the air while you palpate again in the tender area. In patients with normal abdominal musculature the contracted muscles protect the intra-abdominal organs from the compressing fingers. If the tenderness arises from an intra-abdominal organ the tenderness is greatly reduced or eliminated by the tension of the abdominal wall, but if the tenderness arises from the anterior abdominal wall it is unaffected or even exaggerated. This test will fail if the abdominal musculature is very weak or if you are feeling through a diastasis recti.

Cutaneous Hyperesthesia

Another maneuver is to look for cutaneous hyperesthesia. Tenderness arising from the skin is sometimes accompanied by generalized cutaneous hyperesthesia in the area. This is particularly found in radicular neuropathic pain perceived in the abdominal wall. Lightly stroke the skin or the hair with your fingertips or a wisp of cotton and compare corresponding areas on both sides of the abdomen. If you detect a difference in sensitivity this suggests that the tenderness does not arise from an intra-abdominal lesion. One exception to this rule is the cutaneous hyperesthesia that accompanies peritonitis. Such hyperesthesia over the distribution of the right ilioinguinal nerve occurs in some cases of appendicitis.

Rebound Tenderness

Sometimes an area that is tender shows a twinge of greater pain when the finger compressing the area is removed. Such rebound tenderness is a sign of peritoneal irritation. Sometimes one examiner reports rebound tenderness when another does not find it. This discrepancy may be due to defective technique. The defect arises from the way the pressure is released. The examiner should compress the area moderately with one finger, just enough to produce a moderate amount of pain, hold the pressure for a moment or two and then release the pressure very quickly, observing the response of the patient to see if a surge of pain occurs just after the release. The defect arises when the examiner, who is concentrating upon the quickness of the release, in fact "pushes off," giving (unconsciously) a quick increase of pressure in order to facilitate the rapidity of the release. This little push also produces a brief surge of pain, leading him to the false impression of rebound tenderness. You can assure that you do not do this by putting your examining hand in a particular position. You should flex your wrist and extend your finger (either the index finger or the long finger) maximally and then lower your whole hand in this position, moving from your elbow, so that the fully extended finger produces enough compression to produce a moderate but definite degree of pain, and maintain the pressure until the pain has stabilized or subsided. This takes a few seconds. Then release the pressure by flexion of your maximally extended finger and extension of your maximally flexed wrist. With the maximally flexed wrist and maximally extended finger, no "push-off" is possible—only retraction of the finger can occur. Rebound tenderness is evident as a surge of pain that takes up to one second to occur after the quick release. The intensity of the rebound pain is usually much greater than that produced by the pressure itself. The test should be repeated at the primary site and various areas of the abdomen. If the three criteria are met—a momentary delay, an exaggerated intensity at rebound, and reproducibility—rebound tenderness truly exists.

Rebound tenderness probably arises because a viscus, displaced by the compression, moves back to its normal position after release of compression and so rubs up against an inflamed peritoneum. It may occur some distance from the point of compression tenderness. Rebound tenderness may be sharply localized in peritoneal irritation, but is more commonly widespread, since peritonitis generally spreads quickly throughout the peritoneum, there being no major barriers to the spread of the substances that cause it. In localized peritonitis, as may occur in a deep gastric or duodenal ulcer, the peritonitis arises from transmural spread of the inflammation to the visceral peritoneum. Generalized rebound tenderness, indicating widespread peritoneal irritation, strongly suggests a perforated viscus. The tenderness in chemical peritonitis is generally more severe than that in bacterial peritonitis, so that rebound tenderness is an important sign of leakage of pancreatobiliary secretions in perforation of a duodenal ulcer. Bacterial peritonitis, as occurs in colonic perforation or in the spontaneous bacterial peritonitis of cirrhosis, is much less likely to cause generalized rebound tenderness.

The preceding discussion of rebound tenderness is "a long run for a short slide." By that I mean that rebound tenderness is not often a really useful sign. Peritonitis is usually quite evident from rigidity of the abdominal wall, extreme generalized abdominal tenderness, percussion tenderness, or a positive jar test (described later in this chapter as a percussion technique). It is rare indeed that rebound tenderness occurs in the absence of these other signs. They are much gentler to discover. Don't put patients through the painful search for rebound tenderness when you are already quite convinced of the presence of peritoneal irritation.

Referred Tenderness

Sometimes very deep compression in one area of the abdomen produces pain remote from the area of compression. This referred tenderness is easy to understand in terms of the mobility of the viscera. Viscera shift with compression to move or compress the source of tenderness, and so pain occurs in the location of the diseased organ. This is most often demonstrable in inflammation of the bowel in the right lower quadrant (like appendicitis) when compression of the lower quadrant elicits pain in the cecal area because of the shift of gas and fluid in the colon. It can occur with gastric or duodenal ulcers as well, in which case pain is felt in the upper abdomen with lower abdominal compression.

Guarding

Commonly, when tenderness is extreme or superficial, you will feel the abdominal wall muscles become rigid during palpation. This signifies that the patient is guarding himself against pain. The more prompt or extreme the rigidity, the more likely is the source of the pain to be superficial. When the source is in the abdominal wall itself, the rigidity is very prompt and extreme.

Crepitus

Crepitus in the skin with tenderness occurs in some conditions, mainly surgical or accidental trauma, or subcutaneous infection with gas-producing organisms, when gas accumulates beneath the skin. You can feel it as a crackling feeling. You cannot mistake crepitus when you feel it. Gas from trauma or infection is accompanied by tenderness. Gas may migrate to the abdominal wall from the thoracic wall or other parts of the body, or from a fractured rib that has penetrated the lung, in which case there is little or no abdominal tenderness with the crepitus.

Specific Palpation of the Liver Area

In routine examination you should always estimate the liver size, location, consistency, and surface features. First find the caudal border of the right lobe.

This border varies in position according to body habitus as well as disease. In most normal people you can feel the liver edge only in inspiration. It recedes beneath the right costal margin in expiration. In tall people you may not feel it even in very deep inspiration and in short people you may feel it even in expiration. The liver is difficult or impossible to feel in very fat people and in patients with tense ascites. You may sometimes feel the edge of the caudate lobe, a congenital anomaly, to the right of the midline near the costal margin.

To find the liver edge most examiners put the dominant hand, or both hands, with the fingertips apposed, pressed into the abdominal wall and aligned parallel to the anticipated liver edge, or parallel to the rectus inscription (Fig. 10-8). Ask the patient to breathe deeply repeatedly, and move the line of your fingertips cephalocaudad until you feel the liver margin as a moving zone of increased resistance to pressure. Sometimes, when the liver edge is sharp or the liver is rotated anteriorly, you will feel the edge "flip" under your fingertips.

Figure 10-8 also shows an alternative method which is a little quicker, a little more sensitive, and less likely to cause pain when the liver is tender. Appose the fingertips of your dominant hand, curve them slightly, and press them firmly against the abdomen. Align your fingertips at approximately 90° to the line of the anticipated liver margin, with one fingertip pressed against the rib margin. Ask the patient to breath deeply while you move the line of your fingertips first cephalocaudad to find the liver margin and then centrally and laterally to explore the extent of palpability transversely. You can perceive the motion of the liver very easily as it moves from one fingertip to another. You can apply this technique very quickly to explore both lobes of the liver, and the spleen as well.

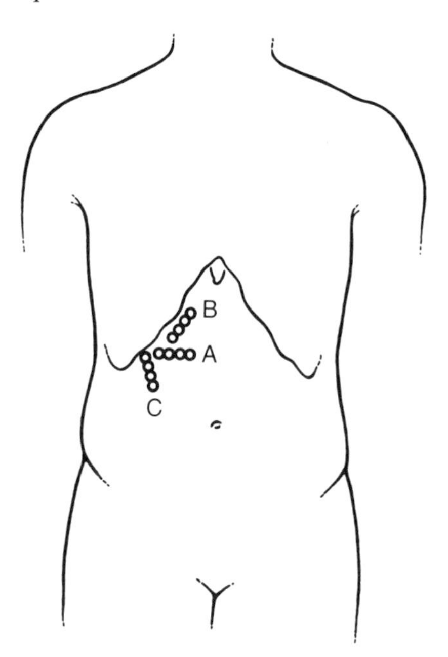

Fig. 10-8. Three ways to align your fingertips in feeling the liver. *A* is the common position. *B* seems somehow less satisfactory. I like *C*, for the reasons explained in the text.

Size

The size of the liver is important to know and changes in size are important to follow. You can express size as the distance of the palpable edge below the costal margin, in the midclavicular line in fixed maximal inspiration, but this measurement is approximate and subject to error, in view of the variability of hepatic accessibility in normal people. It is better to measure *liver span.* You measure this with respect to the right lobe (Fig. 10-9). Determine the position of the caudal margin of the right lobe in the midclavicular line by palpation (or by percussion, if obesity or ascites impedes palpation) with the patient in fixed maximal inspiration. Mark the position with a pen. Then locate the upper surface of the right lobe by percussion of the anterior chest along the midclavicular line. The level of relative hepatic dullness indicates the dome of the right lobe. Mark it with a pen. The distance between the two marks is liver span. Make two or three determinations because the method is not precise. This gives you a reproducible and reasonably faithful estimate of the liver size: 12 cm is about the maximal distance for the normal right hepatic lobe, but it may be greater in very large people and less in those who are very small. In the case of tumors and infiltrative disease, the lobes may be differentially enlarged. That is, the left lobe may be involved and the right lobe spared. This would be suggested by a readily palpable left lobe with a normal span of the right lobe.

Consistency

Note the consistency of the surface of the liver. It is normally smooth, and you can sense this as the surface moves with respiration beneath your fingertips.

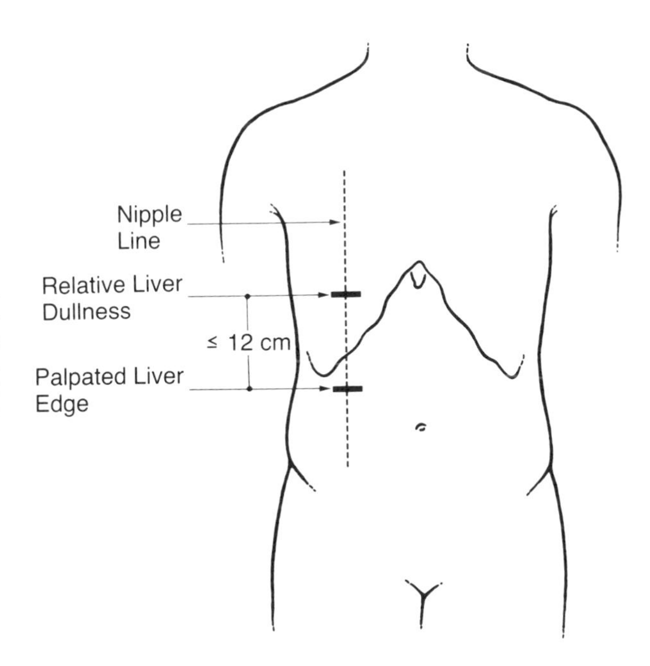

ig. 10-9. The estimation of liver span." The axis upon vhich the measurement is nade is drawn here as the nipple line. Twelve centimeters is he upper limit of normal in dults of average size, but it nay be more or less in very arge or very small people.

The abnormal liver may be nodular, and these nodules may be small (in the "finely nodular liver") larger (in the "coarsely nodular liver"), or massive. Fine nodularity of the liver is almost never perceptible on palpation. You can often detect the coarsely nodular liver. You can usually feel the massively nodular liver to have masses or lumps on the surface, and such a surface is usually described as "irregular"; such gross nodularity is usually more apparent along the edge of the right lobe than on the hepatic surface, and so you should feel carefully all along the liver edge. Massive nodules are either tumors or the regenerative nodules that sometimes occur in cirrhosis.

Firmness

Estimate the firmness of the liver. To know what is normal you need to feel many normal and diseased livers. Even then it can be difficult to be very secure about firmness because of the variability in the amount of fat in the abdominal wall. It is customary to report a normal liver as "soft" and an abnormal liver as "firm" or "hard" (or even "rock hard"). Generalized firmness and hardness imply fibrosis, infiltrative disease, or tumors. Large, widely separated nodules will feel much harder than the hepatic surface between these nodules.

Tenderness

Note the tenderness of the liver. You can usually detect extreme tenderness on light palpation, but the demonstration of less tenderness requires deeper palpation. The normal liver is not tender at all, or only very slightly so. Tenderness occurs in any condition that enlarges the liver, more so when the enlargement is rapid, probably because of the tension exerted on the hepatic capsule. With slow enlargement, the capsule has time to accommodate, and so there is less tenderness. Tenderness is extreme in acute hepatic inflammation (as in hepatitis), much less so in chronic infiltrative disease, hepatic tumors, and cirrhosis. You may find a surprising degree of tenderness in the liver that has enlarged quickly in congestive heart failure. When the size and consistency of the liver surface seem to be normal but the tenderness is extreme, you should suspect inflammation adjacent to the liver, as in subhepatic abscess or gallbladder disease.

The Gallbladder

The gallbladder is small, soft, deep, and closely attached to the liver, so it is usually impossible to distinguish it from the liver on physical examination, even in advanced disease. You will never feel it convincingly as such, except occasionally in advanced carcinoma of the gallbladder, but even then you will almost always interpret it as a liver mass. Only in one condition, hydrops of the gallbladder, can the gallbladder clearly be palpated and even then it is not easy. In hydrops, complete obstruction of the outlet of the gallbladder leads to the accumulation of such large volumes of secreted mucinous fluid that the fundus pushes against the abdominal wall. You can often see this at inspection more easily than you can feel it, but if you see if first you can then sometimes feel it as a smooth rather soft mass, about the size of a ping-pong ball.

Symptomatic gallbladder disease, being usually inflammatory, is more evident as tenderness rather than as a mass. The point of maximal tenderness is over the gallbladder, but the position of the gallbladder is highly variable so this point may be anywhere from close to the midline to close to the anterior axillary line. In those in whom an inflamed tender gallbladder lies above the rib margin, the emergence of the gallbladder in inspiration may cause them to arrest inspiration when the gallbladder descends to encounter your hand compressing the right upper quadrant. The gallbladder is displaced with the liver in hepatomegaly, so the point of maximal tenderness may even be in the right lower quadrant where it may be confused with the tenderness of appendiceal inflammation. If the inflammation of the gallbladder is chronic there may be extension of the inflammation to structures about the gallbladder, like the caudal surface of the right hepatic lobe, in which case the area of the tenderness may be quite large. Tenderness in the gallbladder, like spontaneous pain in the gallbladder, may be projected to the right subscapular region or the lateral supraclavicular area on the right.

Specific Palpation of the Gastric and Duodenal Areas

The epigastrium and the left hypochondrium constitute the gastroduodenal area. You can never convincingly feel the duodenum, and the stomach only rarely in its diseased state. Tenderness is the main finding in disease of this area. You can usually palpate this area adequately with one hand. The critical point is to cover the region with precision.

Tenderness with or without a mass in the gastroduodenal area signifies inflammation. Gastric neoplasms are often not tender but they may be slightly tender if there is significant associated inflammation, as there often is.

When you suspect tenderness in this area from the history or from the survey palpation, you should approach the area from the anticipated margins of the tender area, from the right, left, and below, to discover the exact extent of the tender area. Then, using graded degrees of pressure, explore the area of tenderness to discover the location of the point of maximal tenderness. An efficient way to do this is to use one finger, pressing only enough to produce moderate pain, and pressing with uniform force in a grid-pattern of points over the area. Repeat the procedure several times to assure reproducibility. If you find a single point repeatedly as the point of maximal tenderness, the location of that point suggests the organ of origin. In inflammation limited to the duodenal bulb, this point is at the midline or just to the right of the midline (assuming normal anatomy), about halfway between the umbilicus and the xiphoid process. It may vary considerably in the cephalocaudad line because the position of the duodenum varies. If the point of maximal tenderness is clearly to the left of the midline, the stomach is more likely to be the source of tenderness. If it is exactly in the midline, it may be the duodenal bulb, the pylorus, or the distal antrum.

You should note the extent of the area of tenderness. An uncomplicated duodenal ulcer may produce only a small area of tenderness—1 to 3 cm in diameter, centered to the right of the midline. A bigger area, so centered, suggests transmural spread of the inflammation, sometimes to adjacent viscera. In inflammatory disease of the stomach, the area, usually centered to the left of the midline, is usually much greater because inflammation usually involves more of the stomach. A large area of tenderness over the stomach does not signify transmural spread of the inflammation. Such transmural spread is very uncommon because the gastric wall is so much thicker than the duodenal wall. If pressure in the gastroduodenal area causes pain that radiates into the hypochondrium or toward the umbilicus, you should suspect a more widespread inflammatory process involving adjacent regions, like subhepatic or subdiaphragmatic inflammation, abscess from perforation, or pancreatitis.

Sometimes you will find tenderness in the epigastrium that is centered over the xiphoid process. *Xiphoid tenderness* can be either traumatic or represent a nonspecific form of costochrondritis, and it can produce pain and tenderness in the epigastrium. You can detect this if you gently manipulate the xiphoid process itself. The processes that cause xiphodynia are not often localized specifically to the xiphoid process, and so you can support your suspicion of xiphodynia if you find tenderness when you manipulate the rest of the sternum or the costochondral margins. The *slipping rib* is a common cause of upper abdominal pain or tenderness. It is very easily and commonly missed unless you think of it. The motion of the end of a mobile 10th or 11th rib against an adjacent rib or costal cartilage sets up a traumatic chondritis. You can detect this by finding the mobile rib and reproducing the pain by manipulating it.

You may seek rebound tenderness if there is great epigastric tenderness. Localized rebound tenderness signifies only limited and localized transmural inflammation. Perforation of a gastric or duodenal lesion produces widespread tenderness both to compression and on rebound.

A mass in the gastroduodenal area is much less likely to arise from the stomach or duodenum than from other organs. You may feel the left hepatic lobe and the caudate lobe there; they can be distinguished by their firm consistency and by the fact that they move with respiration, though the motion is less than that of the right hepatic lobe. Duodenal masses are extremely rare and virtually never palpable. You can feel gastric masses (which nearly always represent malignancies) only if they are very large; they show little or no motion with respiration because gastric malignancies that are big enough for you to feel are usually fixed in position. Also, the stomach itself moves little with breathing, being deformable by diaphragmatic movement. You can sometimes feel pancreatic cysts or localized fluid collections in the lesser sac as soft cystic masses in the epigastrium that usually do not move with breathing because of retroperitoneal fixation. Subhepatic or subphrenic abscesses occasionally extend to be palpable in the gastroduodenal area. They do not move with breathing because they tend to be fixed.

Specific Palpation of the Splenic Area

The spleen is the principal organ to feel for in the splenic area. You want to discover its palpability and, if palpable, its characteristics. Any mass or tenderness in this area is abnormal. This is the most difficult of all areas of the abdomen to examine, both because it is far from you when you are at the patient's right side and because you want to feel as far up under the left rib cage as possible.

The simplest way to feel for the spleen is simply to place your dominant hand in the area and to probe gently while the patient breathes deeply. If you feel nothing, you may probe more deeply. In very deep probing, you can use you subordinate hand to press your dominant hand, as described previously.

If you feel nothing and find no tenderness, the maneuvers can be repeated with a pillow or the patient's left fist placed under his left flank or lumbar curvature. This exaggerates the lumbar lordosis and forces deep structures in the left hypochondrium anteriorly making them more accessible. It is also useful for you to put your subordinate hand under the left rib cage and pull it forward. This will displace the spleen forward so that you can feel it with your dominant hand as the patient breathes deeply.

In another important maneuver you place the patient on his right side with his torso flexed and his knees and hips flexed. You then move to the left side of the abdomen, standing behind the patient, and place your hands with your palms against the left costal margin and your fingers arched into the left hypochondrium. In this position the abdominal wall is relaxed and the structures of the splenic fossa fall forward. You probe progressively deeply along the fossa, asking the patient to breath deeply while you hold your fingers in position all along the fossa.

If the clinical history suggests that an enlarged spleen or any other left upper quadrant mass may be present, you should use all of these techniques before you conclude that nothing is palpable in the area.

The motion of the spleen in breathing is very helpful in identifying it. The spleen lies very far to the left and it touches the left diaphragm lateral to the dome. Thus its motion in respiration follows an arcuate path that extends from the intersection of the left midaxillary line with the rib margin toward the umbilicus (Fig. 10-10). This path is very characteristic, and any palpable mass that so moves in deep breathing is either the spleen or something closely attached to it.

The size of the spleen varies enormously. The normal spleen is not palpable. If you can feel it at all, it is almost certainly abnormal. In certain viral infections (like mononucleosis and viral hepatitis) the spleen may protrude only a few centimeters with deep inspiration. The spleen may fill the left upper quadrant when it becomes very large. When that occurs the spleen moves very little with respiration. With such a large immobile mass you may think that it is some mass other than the spleen. You can identify the mass as the spleen by finding the splenic notch, an indentation along the medial border of the mass (Fig. 10-11).

The character of the spleen is highly variable. Its surface nearly always feels

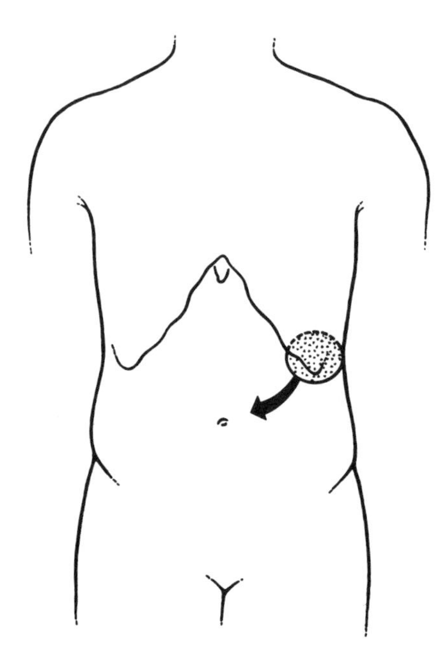

Fig. 10-10. The motion of the spleen in respiration. The arcuate path it follows toward the umbilicus is useful in distinguishing the spleen from other masses in the left upper quadrant. This path is produced by the contact of the spleen with the lateral margin of the left diaphragm.

smooth. Although the spleen may contain nodules, you can rarely feel them. You can usually feel a distinct margin or edge. The firmness of the spleen is highly variable. The degree of firmness is useful in suggesting the cause of splenomegaly. In the splenomegaly that occurs in viral infections the spleen is soft, so soft that it may be difficult for you to distinguish the spleen from the normal contents of the area. It is easier to feel such soft spleens with light

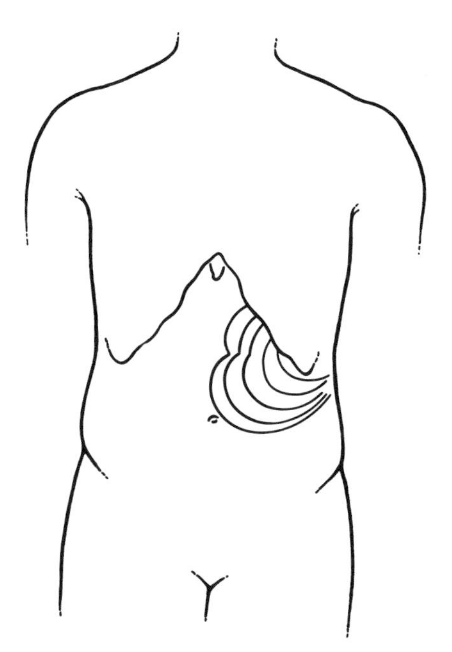

Fig. 10-11. The splenic notch. As the spleen enlarges, its motion with respiration diminishes. With a large mass in the left upper quadrant, the notch on the medial border at the splenic hilum is sometimes helpful to identify the mass as the spleen.

pressure, the motion of a slightly resistant area being more impressive than the palpability of the splenic edge. In infiltrative diseases or other causes of chronic splenomegaly (like cirrhosis, lymphoma, and sarcoid) the spleen is very firm, often approaching the hardness of the cirrhotic liver.

The tenderness of the spleen is variable. It is very tender when the enlargement has been rapid, probably because the splenic capsule has not accommodated. The spleen is also very tender in abscess and infarction. It is only slightly or not at all tender in chronic splenomegaly, probably because the capsule has had time to accommodate.

You may feel other things in the splenic area. A mass in the upper lobe of the left kidney or a suprarenal mass may be confused with the spleen. Such masses usually move little with respiration. If they do, they follow a more craniocaudad path than the spleen does. Since these are usually renal cysts or tumors, they are not very tender. You can mistake an abnormally large left hepatic lobe for the spleen. You can distinguish it by its more craniocaudad path in respiratory motion, by its usually greater firmness, and by its extension to the midline. You can distinguish pancreatic cysts from the spleen by their relative lack of respiratory motion, by their deviation from the characteristic path of splenic motion in respiration, and by the lack of a distinguishably sharp margin. Malignant masses of the stomach or splenic flexure of the colon are sometimes palpable in the splenic area. They can be distinguished from the spleen by their nodularity, by their position a little away from the splenic fossa, and by their relative lack of respiratory motion. Left subphrenic abscesses are very hard to recognize. They may be confused with the spleen and may indeed involve it. They are very tender, do not follow the path of the spleen in respiratory motion, and lack the distinct edge of the spleen.

Specific Palpation of the Umbilical Area

You may palpate the umbilical area either with your dominant hand alone or with pressure from your subordinate hand. Since the lumbar lordotic curvature is maximal in this midline area, the midline retroperitoneal structures lie far forward and are very accessible. Very deep palpation is not necessary. The main structures to consider in the umbilical area are the aorta and the pancreas. Although parts of the small intestine and colon may lie in this region, both organs are highly mobile and any masses that they may contain are likely to slide away to the side of the lumbar protrusion.

It is easy to feel the aorta in thin people, less so in fat people, as an elongated pulsating mass in the midline. Since the aortic bifurcation lies very near the level of the umbilicus, you should feel for the aorta at and cephalad to the umbilicus. Palpability of the aorta may be difficult to interpret. The normal aorta is palpable, especially in old people, because of its elongation and consequent tortuosity. When you think that the aorta is unusually accessible, considering the age and fatness of the patient, you should suspect that there is an aortic aneurysm, the more so if you have heard a bruit. An aneurysm expands laterally with systole while a tortuous aorta does not. You can evaluate systolic lateral expansion of a pulsating mass by pressing the fingers of both your hands deeply into the abdomen with one hand on each side and a few centimeters away from the midline, and then moving them together slightly toward the midline. This is not a highly reliable technique. It is easy to miss even moderately large aneurysms this way. The normal aorta (or something near it) can be moderately tender to palpation, but aneurysms are often distinctly more tender than normal.

It is easy to mistake masses that overlie the aorta for aortic aneurysms because they transmit the systolic pulse to your fingers. There is no sure way to distinguish the two possibilities, but masses that transmit the aortic pulsation are sometimes identifiable as such by nodularity or a distinct edge.

You cannot feel the normal pancreas. The pancreatic head lies cephalad to and well to the right of the umbilicus, and the tail of the pancreas extends to the spleen. The whole organ is retroperitoneal and it is draped over the lumbar curvature, so that the head and tail are too deep to be accessible. Even when the pancreas is greatly enlarged, as in advanced carcinoma, it is rare that you can feel it as a distinct mass. Pancreatic disease is mainly distinguishable at palpation as tenderness. The normal pancreas may be slightly tender. At least many people with a normal pancreas are slightly tender to deep palpation in the area. In the two major diseases of the pancreas—pancreatitis and carcinoma—you may find considerable tenderness, much more so in pancreatitis than in carcinoma. Acute pancreatitis usually leads to exquisite tenderness, often to very light pressure alone or to percussion, that is very diffuse over the whole area. But occasionally there is surprisingly little tenderness in acute pancreatitis. In chronic pancreatitis the pancreas is usually less tender. The usually slight tenderness of pancreatic carcinoma is also quite diffuse, because the cancer often partly obstructs the pancreatic duct and so leads at least to some degree of inflammation throughout the organ.

When you find tenderness in the pancreatic area in a patient with a history that suggests inflammatory pancreatic disease, it is often useful to do the *jar test*. The principle of this test is that the inflamed organ hurts if it is jarred or shaken abruptly. Since the pancreas is fastened to the lumbar spine, any jarring force applied to the lumbar spine shakes the pancreas and induces pain in the area, either or both anteriorly and in the lumbar region. Organs that are suspended by mesenteries do not receive the force that the pancreas does from a jar delivered to the spine. To do the test during the abdominal examination, ask the patient to extend one leg fully and strike his heel with your fist. You should strike very gently at first and then more forcefully, stopping when the anticipated response occurs. Do not tell the patient what response you are looking for, but only ask if the blow produces any discomfort. In most cases of acute pancreatitis, there is no doubt of a positive response: The pain may be severe, though momentary. If there is a positive response, you should ask the patient about its location and its resemblance to the abdominal pain that he had complained of. You can do the same test with the patient standing, asking him to rise on his toes and drop suddenly on his heels. This is much less satisfactory, since you do not control the force of the blow. A positive jar test most commonly represents pancreatitis, but it is not specific for pain of pancreatic origin. It is positive in pain originating from any retroperitoneal structure fixed to the spine or from the spine itself. It is also positive in peritonitis, where the response is more generalized. The test may be negative in minor or resolving cases of pancreatitis.

Pancreatic cysts often appear as masses in the pancreatic area. You should suspect them if you feel a moderately tender mass that is globular, lacks a sharp edge, and is fixed in position.

Specific Palpation of the Renal Areas

Since structures in the flanks are deep, you must pull them forward with your subordinate hand while you feel with your dominant hand through the anterior abdominal wall. Because the motion of a mass helps you to feel it, you move your subordinate hand forward to press the viscera against your stationary dominant hand. There is little to feel in the flanks except for the kidneys and the colon.

The normal kidneys are usually not palpable except in very slender people, but when you feel a mass in either flank it is far more likely to be the kidney than anything else. You can move the normal kidney rather freely. It may move caudad to some degree when the patient breathes deeply, but this varies. Respiratory motion of the kidneys may be increased if there is a large spleen or liver to transmit diaphragmatic motion to the kidneys. Even with a very large kidney or a kidney containing a very large mass, it is hard to feel a distinct lateral edge because of the rounded contour of the organ and the overlying fat in the flanks. You can almost never feel a distinct medial margin because of the depth of the organ and the thickness of the viscera and fat. The size of a kidney cannot be accurately measured because of this obscurity of its margins. The kidneys usually feel smooth, but large polycystic kidneys may feel nodular. If you feel a mobile smooth mass in the flank of a patient of normal or increased corpulence, you should suspect it to be an enlarged kidney.

The normal kidney is a little tender. Inflammatory masses are exquisitely tender while neoplastic masses are not. Renal tumors are more likely to be felt anteriorly, and perinephric abscesses posteriorly. The kidney that is enlarged because of outlet obstruction is not very tender. You may feel a perinephric abscess as a very tender mass that does not move with respiration.

The firmness of the normal kidney is about the same as that of the normal liver. You can almost never appreciate the increased firmness of a renal tumor or the resilience of a renal cyst or an obstructed kidney.

You may feel other things in the renal areas. Apart from the kidneys, other masses in the flanks are nearly always colonic tumors. When they are palpable at all, you feel them as anterior because they are intraperitoneal rather than retroperitoneal. They are usually rather mobile since the colon is mobile, unless they are very large and sufficiently advanced to have become attached to the posterior wall of the abdomen. They are commonly nodular. They are often moderately tender because they are usually associated with some local inflammation.

Specific Palpation of the Lower Quadrants

In the right lower quadrant you are feeling mainly for the terminal ileum, the cecum, and the ascending colon, and for the descending colon in the left. The fossae are deep. Masses in the fossae are difficult to reach and their edges are hard to define.

You should use your dominant hand alone for light or moderately deep palpation in these areas. For very deep palpation, you can use your subordinate hand to press your dominant hand into the abdomen. The structures in these areas vary in position and are mobile. You should first palpate lightly over the whole region with two or three fingers applied in a grid-pattern, noting areas of tenderness and resistance. You can then repeat this with slightly deeper palpation. Whether or not you find masses or tenderness at this point, you should repeat the procedure with progressively deeper palpation, moving the fingers slightly mediolaterally at each point of compression. Because masses here are nearly always mobile, you can more easily feel a mass as it rolls under your examining fingers than you can by its resistance to stationary compression.

Most masses in the iliac fossae arise from the intestine and colon. The normal cecum is sometimes mistaken for a mass. Masses are not usually palpable until they have become quite large. The absence of a palpable mass never excludes a mass lesion in a patient who has suggestive symptoms. You should gauge the smoothness of a mass. The nodularity of a malignant mass may be perceptible. Inflammatory masses do not often feel nodular. Note the firmness of the mass. Malignant masses are very hard while inflammatory masses often have a firmness like that of the normal liver. You cannot feel a localized abscess itself as a mass because its softness does not allow it to be distinguished from normal tissue. What you feel is the indurated mesentery or the adherent bowel. Inflammatory masses are always tender, malignant masses much less so.

You may feel other masses in the lower quadrants. It is easy to mistake a distended urinary bladder for a pathologic mass in a patient who has urinary retention. A distended bladder is symmetrical, globular, and in the midline, extending as far as the umbilicus in the most extreme cases, with a soft to firm character and slight to moderate tenderness. You can identify it as the bladder by its disappearance after voiding or catheterization. You may feel gross enlargement of the uterus or adnexal structures in the lower quadrants. Their confirmation as such must be made at a bimanual pelvic examination. It is common to confuse feces in the colon for a pathologic mass in constipated patients. You can often feel feces in the left lower quadrant in normal people. You will not often feel feces in the right lower quadrant because feces in the right colon is usually fluid. You can recognize fecal masses by their smoothness and plasticity, location, mobility, and lack of tenderness.

Tenderness without a mass is common in both lower quadrants. The normal colon is slightly tender in some people, especially in the left lower quadrant. Deciding if the tenderness is abnormal on direct compression alone requires experience and judgment.

Percussion of the Abdomen

The Purpose and Technique of Percussion

Palpation will tell you most of what you can find in the abdomen before you percuss. Percussion is useful for a few specific purposes: to find ascites, to measure organs or distended viscera, and to explore tenderness when it is too severe to be explored by palpation.

Tap the abdominal wall with one or two fingers of your dominant hand, using a finger of the subordinate hand as a pleximeter. As in the cardiac examination, deliver taps at points along a straight line moving from resonant areas into the areas expected to show dullness.

Most of the abdomen resonates because most of the abdomen contains gas-filled intestine. You will encounter dullness only when fluid or solid organs or masses directly contact the abdominal wall. Thus, for example, a liver that is palpable may not be detected by percussion, if, as occasionally happens, a segment of colon is interposed between the liver and the abdominal wall.

Generalized Abdominal Percussion

Gas in the bowel gives a slight resonance to the normal abdomen so that normal resonance extends only to the level in the flanks where structures without gas lie beneath the abdominal wall. When much of the bowel is distended with gas, the abdomen is hyperresonant. The resonant note is higher in pitch and more "musical" than usual. This is hard to judge, and it is reliable as an indicator of gaseous bowel distension only when it is extreme.

Generalized abdominal percussion is most useful in finding ascites. The two techniques that are used are the search for *shifting dullness* and the search for a *fluid wave.* These are not, in fact, very useful signs in finding small degrees of ascites.

In seeking shifting dullness, you seek to find if the level of dullness in the flanks shifts when you rotate the body of the patient. With the patient supine you percuss along a transverse line from the umbilicus into the flank to establish (and mark) the level of dullness that signifies the lower extent of bowel. Then rotate the patient 45° to 90° toward the side of the flank that you are examining. After a few moments, repeat percussion along the same line. Mark the level of dullness in the flank again. If the level does not change, ascites has not been demonstrated; if ascites is present, the level shifts toward the umbilicus (Fig. 10-12). You should repeat the test several times in both flanks. The level shifts because gas-filled bowel floats upward in the peritoneal fluid (Fig. 10-13). It may take several moments for this shifting to occur, so allow a little time between the first and second stages. The test is rather insensitive. It does not reveal small degrees of ascites. It is sometimes not positive in massive (or "tense") ascites because the bowel is so crowded that it cannot float. It works best in finding moderate degrees of ascites.

You can also seek a fluid wave when you suspect ascites. The term refers to

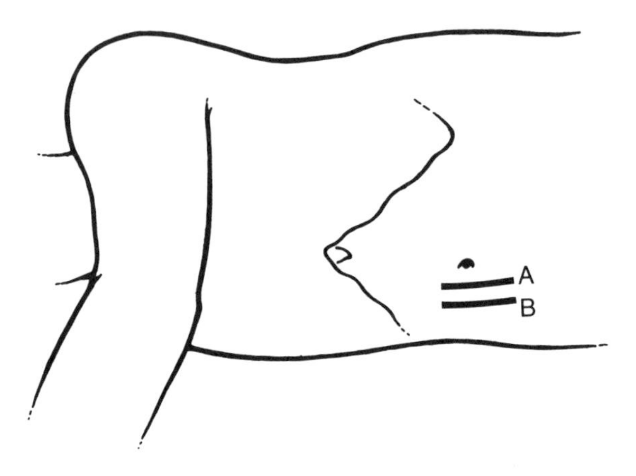

Fig. 10-12. Shifting dullness. The level of dullness shifts toward the umbilicus (from *B* to *A*) as the patient is rotated from supine to lateral recumbency.

the fact that when you tap the surface of an elastic closed vessel containing an incompressible fluid, you can feel the wave of motion in the fluid at other points on the surface of the vessel. The normal abdomen contains both gas and fluid, but the fluid is normally separated into compartments by gas. Because gas is compressible and fluid is not, induced fluid wave motion is not transmitted

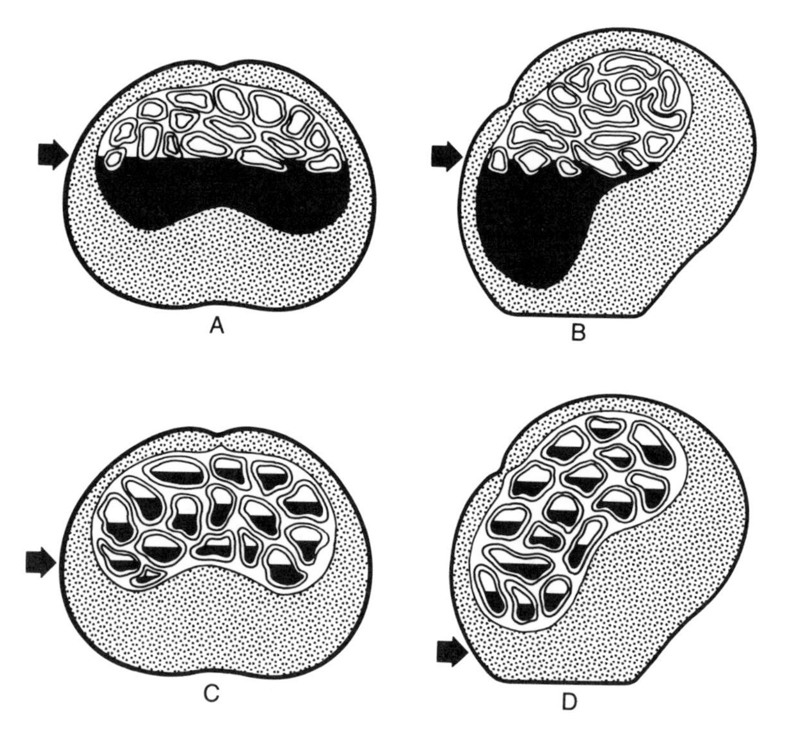

Fig. 10-13. Why ascites produces shifting dullness while fluid-filled bowel does not. (**A & B**) The ascitic fluid forms a level which shifts as the patient is rotated laterally. (**C & D**) Although the fluid levels shift in the bowel compartments, no change in the level of flank dullness occurs.

through the normal abdomen. A fluid wave is transmitted when there is a continuous fluid mass from one side of the abdomen to the other. You press the palmar surfaces of the fingers of your examining hand into one flank and tap at the other flank sharply and forcefully with the fingers of your other hand. Press the ulnar margin of a third hand (which can be that of the patient) firmly into the abdomen along the midline at the level of the umbilicus to dampen wave transmission through the abdominal wall. You will feel a fluid wave as a distinct pulse following the tap, with a distinct delay, something less than a second. You should repeat the test several times in both directions (right to left, left to right) to determine its reproducibility. Like shifting dullness, the fluid wave does not detect small degrees of ascites. It is distinct only in massive ascites.

Another method to find a small amount of ascites is to seek the *puddle sign.* Have the patient lie prone for 5 minutes and then have him rise to his elbows and knees. You put your stethoscope to the midline at the most dependent point of the abdomen and begin tapping or flicking with a consistent force in the patient's flank on the side toward you. You move your stethoscope diaphragm away from the midline to the far side of the abdomen while you flick constantly in the same place. When the diaphragm of the stethoscope reaches the far side of a puddle of ascitic fluid, the sound produced by the flicking becomes louder. This technique is good to detect small quantities of ascites, but it requires that the patient be able to get into and hold the proper position, and it is awkward to perform.

Percussion of the Liver and Spleen

Sometimes you cannot feel the liver or an enlarged spleen because of fat, fluid, or gas. If these organs lie against the abdominal wall, you can find their margins by percussion. Percuss in a straight line moving from an area of resonance at a right angle to the margin of the anticipated area of dullness.

When massive ascites impedes palpation of the liver and spleen, the dullness of the ascitic fluid relative to that of gas-filled bowel may make it impossible to find these organs by percussion. In that case a form of *ballottement* is useful. This technique takes advantage of the fact that these movable organs are suspended within the ascitic fluid mass, not floating at the surface, because they have about the same specific gravity as ascitic fluid. The organs may not be palpable because they are easily displaced into the yielding fluid volume. You tap very forcefully over the organ leaving your fingers pressed firmly at the point where the tap was delivered. You can feel the organ bounce back against the abdominal wall after a slight delay. By doing this over a large area, you can get some impression of the size and firmness of the organ.

Percussion for Tenderness

When an organ or region is so tender that even light palpation is intolerable, you can use percussion to map the area of tenderness. Light taps are effective in eliciting tenderness in this situation, and they produce only momentary pain.

You can also use percussion to define tenderness in regions that are inaccessible to palpation, the splenic and hepatic fossae and in the lumbar regions. This requires the use of *fist percussion,* in which you use one hand flattened against the body wall as a pleximeter and the fist of the other as a hammer. You should tap very gently at first and then repeat the taps with increasing force until you are satisfied about the presence or absence of tenderness. Fist percussion is a form of jar-percussion. The motion produced by the shaking of an acutely enlarged or inflamed organ is painful. Tenderness to fist percussion over the right lower rib cage occurs in many conditions. You should use the method with great caution, and only when you suspect tenderness in the area and do not detect it by palpation. Pain produced by fist percussion can be very severe; remember that a sharp blow produces far more pain than gentle palpation does. You tend to lose your appreciation of force when you tap with your fist.

Some Special Tests to Find Retroperitoneal Extension of Lower Abdominal Infections, like Appendicitis

In appendicitis, regional enteritis, and diverticulitis, the inflammatory process occasionally extends to involve the adjacent retroperitoneal muscles in the pelvis. You can usually tell that such extension has occurred because the patient has pain in the region when he walks, or because he lies holding his leg still, usually flexed. If the process is milder, you can detect it by stretching or tensing these muscles.

In the *iliopsoas test* you ask the supine patient to keep his knee extended and to raise his thigh against the pressure that you exert against the thigh with your hand. If the iliopsoas muscle is inflamed, the maneuver produces pain in the pelvis. You can do the same thing by hyperextending the leg at the hip with the patient lying on his side. This form of the test is sometimes positive in mild inflammation of the muscle when the iliopsoas test performed with the patient supine is equivocal.

In the *obturator test,* you ask the supine patient to flex his hip and thigh to 90°. You fix his knee by holding his leg with one hand on the calf and the other on the thigh, and you rotate the leg medially. If the obturator muscle is inflamed, this maneuver produces pain in the pelvis.

These are classical tests used in the diagnosis of acute appendicitis. I have seen positive tests in either leg in regional enteritis, and in the left leg in colonic diverticulitis. These signs are rarely primary or major physical manifestations of these diseases, but they provide helpful supportive evidence for them if the more usual manifestations—pain, fever, ileus, and altered bowel habit—are mild or equivocal.

These maneuvers can produce extreme pain when the muscle is very severely involved. Do not do them if the involvement is obvious; if you do them, be slow and gentle as you proceed.

THE ANAL AND RECTAL EXAMINATION

The Position of the Patient

You can best examine the anus and rectum with the patient in the knee–chest position in bed or on a sigmoidoscopy table, or bent over the examination table. You can do digital examination with the patient lying or standing. Perianal inspection is less satisfactory in those positions. A really thorough examination requires examination in several positions.

Inspection of the Perianal Area

The perianal skin is normally slightly hyperpigmented for a variable distance around the anal opening. Pigmentation is enhanced after healing of superficial inflammation like intertrigo. Abrasions in the area are common in pruritus ani.

You sometimes see *perianal openings.* It is common to see the opening of a pilonidal sinus in the posterior midline near the tip of coccyx. The opening may be surrounded by inflamed skin. Any other opening in the area is likely to be the external opening of a fistula in ano. Fistulous openings occur at variable distances from the anus and in any quadrant. Those that are posterior to the midline usually communicate to the posterior rectal wall and those anterior to this line communicate to the anterior wall. Fistulous openings very close to the anus usually communicate to the anterior rectal wall. The external openings are usually surrounded by a zone of inflammation, and they sometimes discharge purulent or feculent fluid with perianal compression. When fistulas are indolent and chronic, have been treated by sitz baths, or lie close to the anal canal, the inflammation may be so slight that perianal hyperpigmentation obscures the openings, or they may be buried in the skin folds that radiate to the anal canal. You must spread the perianal skin to look for them.

Visible perianal masses are common. A mass over the coccyx in the posterior midline is a pilonidal cyst. Genital warts occur in any perianal quadrant and at a variable distance from the anal opening. They are usually multiple, highly variable in size, nodular, and sometimes hyperpigmented. They feel firm. Skin tags are usually solitary, though there may be two or three. They are irregular pliable masses, rarely more than about 5 mm in diameter, that lie adjacent to the anal canal, commonly at the end of a radiating fold of perianal skin. They are smooth and have the color of the normal skin. They feel soft. External hemorrhoids look much like skin tags, having a similar position and appearance except for color. If you have your patient strain, you can often recognize an external hemorrhoid as it is engorged with blood and everted. Occasionally, you will see an enlarged anal papilla, especially if you have the patient strain. The papilla, normally only about 1 to 2 mm in diameter, may be everted as a pink-white mass, up to 1.5 cm in diameter, smooth, firm, and triangular. Carcinomas of the anal canal are usually visible as nodular firm masses.

Fissures in the anal canal often extend externally far enough for you to see them. Spread the perianal skin to flatten the radiating folds. A fissure will appear as a bright pink or pink-white crack in the depth of one such fold, extending into the depth of the anal opening. It can be painful to expose it in this way.

During inspection of the perianal region, you should always ask the patient to strain in order to reveal external hemorrhoids or enlarged papillae. This may also reveal rectal prolapse. You may not detect mild degrees of rectal prolapse when the patient strains in the knee–chest position or lying on his side. Prolapse is sometimes evident only when he is seated. If you strongly suspect prolapse, have him strain when he is squatting or seated on a commode that allows you to look at his perineum.

Digital Examination

You palpate the anal canal and rectum to find things that you cannot see. It is convenient to do this with the patient in the knee–chest position, preferably on a sigmoidoscopy table, as a part of perianal inspection and sigmoidoscopic examination. You can reach farther and you feel the anterior rectal wall better in the knee–chest position. You can feel the posterior rectal wall better with the patient supine or lying on his side. In a truly thorough palpation, you should do a digital examination in both positions.

Coat your gloved finger with lubricant and apply lubricant liberally to the anal opening. Insert your finger very slowly so as not to provoke a reactive spasm of the anal sphincter. When the anal canal seems very tender, use an anesthetic gel as a lubricant and use your little finger rather than your index finger.

At first insert your finger only far enough to feel the inner margin of the anal canal with the pad of your fingertip. Then press gently, feeling in all quadrants. Note the resistance to pressure as an estimate of sphincter tone. Ask the patient to squeeze hard. The increased force you feel comes from contraction of the external sphincter, which is voluntary, while the force you feel when the patient is not squeezing comes from the internal sphincter, which is involuntary. In this way you can estimate the strength of the two sphincters separately. Ask the patient about tenderness at each location where you press. This helps you to locate a fissure that was not apparent externally. Note any masses that you feel in the anal canal. The normal anal canal is symmetrical and smooth. Hemorrhoids are not usually palpable but they may be if they are thrombotic. Enlarged papillae are not palpable. You should always consider a hard mass in the anal canal to be malignant. A stricture is palpable as a symmetrical narrowing that does not yield to the finger. Do not try to force past a stricture, as it can be very painful to the patient.

Then insert your finger fully to feel the rectal wall in all quadrants. You should be able to feel the coccyx posteriorly, and the prostate or cervix anteriorly. You should use these as landmarks in describing other masses or areas of tenderness. You may feel a pararectal abscess as a tender fluctuant mass laterally.

Carcinomas feel like circumferential hard narrowings. Occasionally you may feel a hard extraluminal mass anteriorly at the end of your fully inserted finger, the *rectal shelf,* representing pelvic metastasis of an intra-abdominal malignancy. Adnexal masses may be palpable laterally if they are very large.

The Sigmoidoscopic and Anoscopic Examinations

How to do the Examination

The fact that the conventional rigid instrument is called a sigmoidoscope is misleading. It cannot permit visualization of the whole sigmoid colon. Sigmoidoscopy (or proctoscopy) allows you to inspect mainly the rectum and the anal canal. Anoscopy with the beveled or slotted anoscope needs to be done separately only when you strongly suspect anal canal disease.

The examination is often flawed because certain points in technique are neglected. The position of the patient is the most important feature of the technique. Sigmoidoscopy is best done with the patient in the knee–chest position on a sigmoidoscopy table. With the patient in any other circumstances, the sigmoidoscopic examination is more difficult and less complete. To assure the easiest and most thorough examination, you should observe the following general points:

1. Get the patient in the right position at the outset. The weight of the patient should be supported entirely on the knees and upper chest. Be sure that the abdominal wall is suspended some distance above the surface of the sigmoidoscopy table and that it is relaxed. This position requires that the knee support of the table be high enough. Ask the patient to kneel on the knee support and rest his chest on the table. Have the shoulder or head support in such a position on the table that his thighs are vertical. Ask the patient to sway his back. Many patients will quickly assume the correct position if you ask them to "lie like a baby who is sleeping with his bottom up in the air." When the hips are elevated and the abdomen and spine are relaxed, the abdominal wall and viscera fall toward the table top and this allows air to flow into the rectum when the sigmoidoscope is inserted.

2. Stand at the side of the patient's buttocks, not directly behind. Stand with your subordinate hand next to the patient. Place the forearm of your subordinate hand on the patient's sacrum, using that hand to hold and control the sigmoidoscope. This leaves your dominant hand free to handle the suction tip, biopsy forceps, and sponges. It also means that the sigmoidoscope does not wave around as you move because you are holding it with a hand that is braced on the sacrum.

3. When you are prepared to insert the instrument, be sure that you have first prepared the anal canal. You should have done digital examination first to lubricate the canal, to dilate the sphincter, and to discover anything that you particularly want to look at.

4. Insert the instrument as slowly as you inserted your finger, and be sure

that you aim it toward the umbilicus until the tip has passed through the anal canal. Then remove the obturator and look as you angle the tip toward the sacrum.

5. Use the air-bulb with hesitancy. You will not need it in slender relaxed patients who are properly positioned. In obese people who cannot get the abdominal wall off the table, or in tense people, inflate the rectum sparingly as necessary.

6. Do not consider it your professional duty to pass the instrument to the hilt. Few patients can tolerate straightening of the sigmoid colon. Pass the instrument only to the point where definite discomfort occurs or else you will not be allowed to do the examination again.

7. Although you may note abnormalities as you advance the instrument, make your principal examination by rotating the instrument as you withdraw it.

8. Do not neglect the anal canal. You can usually see it quite well with the sigmoidoscope if you withdraw it "1 mm at a time." You do not need to use the anoscope except in special circumstances. When you feel you must see the anal canal better, use the slotted or beveled anoscope, inserting it repeatedly to examine each quadrant. Do not rotate the anoscope with the obturator removed. If you probe crevices in the anal canal to find fissures or infected crypts, be very cautious. The inflamed squamous epithelium is very tender.

9. Talk to your patient during the whole examination. Tell him what you are going to do in advance. Tell him what you are doing as you do it. Tell him what you saw when you are finished. When you talk you help to keep the patient relaxed. This is a very important use of "verbal anesthesia."

What to Look For in Sigmoidoscopy and Anoscopy

Subtle mucosal inflammation is the most difficult thing to recognize at sigmoidoscopy. Intense inflammation is easy to recognize, but inflammation may be subtle early in the course of inflammatory disease and in healing inflammation.

The clarity of the vasculature is the feature of the mucosa that is most susceptible to change in mild inflammation. You can clearly see submucosal vessels in the normal rectum. These include large veins that bulge slightly into the lumen and arborized veins that are flat. They are most conspicuous in the rectal ampulla and between the rectal valves. The anal canal does not contain prominent vessels other than hemorrhoids, nor are vessels prominent over the rectal valves. Even slight mucosal edema obscures submucosal vessels. It is easy to overlook such obscurity. You must always make a particularly conscious effort to evaluate the distinctness of the submucosal vessels.

Blunting of the rectal valves is another subtle sign of mucosal edema. The normal valve has a finely wrinkled surface and a sharp edge. In mucosal edema the surface is smoother and the edges have a rounded appearance.

The *normal mucosal surface texture* is smooth and shiny. In mucosal edema the surface has a granular appearance or appears to be "dry" so that it does not glisten.

You should assess *mucosal friability* when you suspect subtle inflammation. The normal mucosa does not bleed when it is rubbed gently with a moistened cotton swab. In subtle inflammation a gentle rub with a moistened cotton swab produces punctate bleeding in the area that was rubbed. Be sure to look for blood on the swab too.

More severe inflammation of the mucosa is readily evident as erythema, intramucosal hemorrhage, exudate, or ulceration. These offer no problems in recognition.

You will occasionally mistake a localized hemorrhage in the anterior rectal wall produced by an enema nozzle tip for an area of inflammation. You can often see such an abrasion in patients who have had a preparatory enema. The adjacent mucosa will appear to be normal. The usual enemas used in preparation for sigmoidoscopy can produce some erythema and some slight obscurity of vessels. They do not affect mucosal friability or texture. Enemas are usually not necessary to prepare for examination in cases where you strongly suspect inflammation of the mucosa since the rectum usually contains so little stool that you can see much of the mucosa adequately. Stool may, of course, hide polyps and malignancies.

You must biopsy any mass lesion and any inflammation, localized or generalized. According to conventional practice, you should delay a barium enema after biopsy of the rectum until time for healing has elapsed, 1 to 3 weeks according to various opinions, because of the danger of perforation or submucosal dissection of the contrast medium. If a lesion is present and you plan to do a barium enema examination, defer biopsy until after the barium enema is done.

When a circumscribed lesion is present you should take at least four biopsies from its margins. In the case of generalized mucosal inflammation, it is best to take biopsies from the edges of the rectal valves. Biopsy at this site is technically easier, you obtain a larger sample, and problematical bleeding is less likely to occur.

In the anal canal, hemorrhoids are engorged veins that extend above the pectinate line (internal hemorrhoids) or below it (external hemorrhoids). Hemorrhoids usually accompany local infection, and so you may also see an infected papilla enlarged by edema. It is a large, pale, triangular mass below the pectinate line. Learn what normal papillae look like—small pink triangles pointing toward the lumen—so that you can recognize the enlarged papillae of papillitis. An enlarged papilla usually has an infected crypt next to it. In cryptitis, the crypts are redder than normal and often contain a little pus. When you see such evidence of infection, especially when there is much anal tenderness, look for a fissure by gently spreading the anal mucosa to see if you can see the characteristic deep red streak, often with a white base.

SUGGESTED READINGS

Davenport H: Physiology of the Digestive Tract, 5th Ed. Year Book Medical Publishers, Chicago, 1982

DeGowin EL, DeGowin RL: Bedside Diagnostic Examination, 4th Ed. Macmillan, New York 1981

Engel GL, Morgan WL (eds): Interviewing the Patient. WB Saunders, Philadelphia, 1973

Gelin-L-E, Nyhus LM, Condon RE (eds): Abdominal Pain: A Guide to Rapid Diagnosis. JB Lippincott, Philadelphia, 1969

Granger DN, Barrowman JA, Kvietys PR: Clinical Gastrointestinal Physiology. WB Saunders, Philadelphia, 1985

Greenberger NJ (ed): Gastrointestinal Disorders: A Pathophysiologic Approach. 3rd Ed. Year Book Medical Publishers, Chicago, 1986

Johnson L: Gastrointestinal Physiology, 3rd Ed. CV Mosby, St. Louis, 1985

Judge RD, Zuidema GD (eds): Clinical Diagnosis: A Physiologic Approach, 4th Ed. Little, Brown & Co, 1982

Silen W: Cope's Early Diagnosis of the Acute Abdomen. 16th Ed. Oxford University Press, New York, 1983

INDEX

Page numbers followed by f represent figures; page numbers followed by t represent tables.

A

B

G

H

I

J

P

R

S